PRAISE FOR
THE WELL-LIVED LIFE

"Dr. Gladys is a global pioneer who has helped transform our very definition of health and healing. Her extraordinary book will offer millions of readers the simple yet revolutionary secrets to discover true health and happiness at any age."

—Mark Hyman, *New York Times* bestselling author of *Young Forever* and *The Pegan Diet*

"Dr. Gladys McGarey is the true mother of holistic medicine, a visionary and pioneer who at the age of 103 is still sharing her wisdom with all of us. As founder of the American Holistic Medical Association, she has taught clinicians a different and more powerful path to healing. I stand witness to her love of people everywhere and have been honored to watch her make the world a better place."

—Mimi Guarneri, MD, FACC, president of the Academy of Integrative Health and Medicine, director of Guarneri Integrative Health

"You will love the stories, you will learn how to honor your health and your body, and in the end, you'll love life that much more. Dr. Gladys's life and work are an incredible example of ever greater joy and fulfillment as we continue to learn and age into our soul's true purpose. She writes one of those rare gems of a story that teaches as much as it inspires."

—Edith Eger, *New York Times* bestselling author of *The Choice* and *The Gift*

"In this age of quick fixes and simplistic solutions to life's problems, Gladys McGarey's approach is just what the doctor ordered. Dr. McGarey speaks to rich and complex truths that will resonate with readers' hearts and minds. She inhabits the real world, where body, brain, and spirit are inseparable, and her century of wisdom is infused with science, medicine, and soul."

—Dr. Robert Waldinger, director of the Harvard Study
of Adult Development and author of *The Good Life*

"Dr. Gladys is as illuminating as she is engaging. Her important work reveals how each of us can live our healthiest and happiest life by connecting with our true purpose. Her combination of medical knowledge and lived experience will be an empowering guide for legions."

—Sara Gottfried, MD, *New York Times* bestselling
author of *Women, Food, and Hormones*

"A brilliant and funny friend, Dr. Gladys lives and shares an extraordinary life filled with curiosity, love, and laughter. She is an international treasure, a pioneer in holistic medicine, who for many decades has described and promoted many methods for preventing and treating illness at home. In this book, published after her 103rd birthday, our lives are further blessed by the light of her kindness and wisdom."

—Dr. Ali Gabriel, DrPH, MS, CST-D

"*The Well-Lived Life* is refreshingly simple and practical. The good doctor's sound advice feels achievable, and readers will feel inspired and energized."

—*Booklist*

The Well-Lived Life

A 103-YEAR-OLD DOCTOR'S
SIX SECRETS TO HEALTH AND
HAPPINESS AT EVERY AGE

GLADYS McGAREY, MD

ATRIA PAPERBACK
New York • London • Toronto • Sydney • New Delhi

ATRIA
PAPERBACK

An Imprint of Simon & Schuster, LLC
1230 Avenue of the Americas
New York, NY 10020

First Atria Paperback edition April 2024

ATRIA PAPERBACK and colophon are trademarks of Simon & Schuster, LLC

Simon & Schuster: Celebrating 100 Years of Publishing in 2024

For information about special discounts for bulk purchases,
please contact Simon & Schuster Special Sales at 1-866-506-1949
or business@simonandschuster.com.

The Simon & Schuster Speakers Bureau can bring authors to your live event.
For more information or to book an event, contact the Simon & Schuster Speakers
Bureau at 1-866-248-3049 or visit our website at www.simonspeakers.com.

Interior design by Dana Sloan

Manufactured in the United States of America

5 7 9 10 8 6

Library of Congress Control Number: 2022951729

ISBN 978-1-6680-1448-6
ISBN 978-1-6680-1449-3 (pbk)
ISBN 978-1-6680-1450-9 (ebook)

To five generations of love and healing in my family, and to you, my reader, may you find that these words help heal your body and guide your soul. You are here for a reason.

CONTENTS

Over the course of eight decades in medicine and ten on the planet, I've worked with thousands of people. I've included many of their stories here, as best as I can remember them. In the interest of privacy, I've changed many of their names, shifted crucial details in their stories, and in some cases combined several people's experiences into one. What I haven't changed is the profound soul transformation I witnessed in them and the equally profound effect each of them has had on my own soul's path.

FOREWORD

_____

Mark Hyman, MD

When I first met Dr. Gladys, I knew I was encountering one of the great healers and wise elders of our time. Countless others have had the same reaction when meeting her. One has the sense that this is a person who has a profound understanding of the human condition—its joys and its sorrows, its inevitable struggles and its savored celebrations. She's a natural healer with an uncommon warmth and hard-earned wisdom. Meeting Dr. Gladys in these pages is no different. Her first popular book is over a hundred years in the making, and it was worth the wait. Dr. Gladys is a global pioneer who has helped transform our very definition of health and healing. Her extraordinary book will offer millions of readers the simple yet revolutionary secrets to discover true health and happiness at any age.

Dr. Gladys has spent nearly eighty years in the medical field—or more, if you count her unofficial training in assisting her medical missionary parents as they tended to some of the most vulnerable and disenfranchised patients in India. Dr. Gladys has long been known as the mother of holistic medicine, although "grandmother" or perhaps "great-grandmother" would be more accurate now. After training as a doctor during World War II, facing significant sexism as one of the pioneering women in the field, she went on to form the American Holistic Medical Association in 1978 as the only female founding member. Her boundless curiosity in exploring effective alternative practices led her to study a range of healing methods from Western, Eastern, and Indigenous cultures and apply them to her practice, long before such an approach was practiced by other physicians. Her belief in honoring mothers and demedicalizing natural processes led her to champion safe home births throughout the 1960s and 1970s. Dr. Gladys was also an early advocate of nutrition in the allopathic field, realizing that what we eat affects every cell in our body—an understanding that has had an important influence on generations of doctors. Finally, her belief that our illnesses can offer us insight into our lives and our souls' growth remains radical in the medical field.

The Well-Lived Life will become a classic not just for generations of patients and practitioners, but also for people who are simply longing for a richer and happier life. Like Dr. Gladys herself, it seems to speak as much to the aches of the soul as to those of the body. This book explores the deepest source of where illness and health, dis-ease and well-being originate. The healing she advocates for is as much spiritual as physical. Dr. Gladys explains that true health is about transforming our relationship with life's inevitable challenges, suffering, and illnesses so that we can experience profound joy and fulfillment.

Providing a road map for how to experience all that life has to offer, Dr. Gladys models everything she teaches. She gives readers a shining example of life as it is meant to be experienced: as a moving, evolving process where we spend our energy wildly and "age into health." In a world that is often anti-aging, Dr. Gladys offers us a positive vision of what our inevitable march of years can become—a source of ever greater joy and fulfillment as we continue to learn and fulfill our soul's true purpose. In other words, how we can live our best life in every moment, so that when our days come to their eventual end, we can know they were truly well-lived.

Dr. Gladys's six secrets are brought to life by her inspiring personal stories and those of her patients, many of whom experience truly miraculous healing. Her patients don't just heal their diseases, they heal their lives. This book is the culmination of everything Dr. Gladys has learned and taught for a century. And while many may consider her life well-lived, it's worth noting that she's not done living it yet. Dr. Gladys lives a more active life than many half her age, and she still has a ten-year plan. As she proudly states, at 103, she's just getting started.

Introduction

TOWARD LIFE

I turned 103 this year. As a doctor in her second century, I am often asked the secret of a long, healthy, happy life. Do I run? Do Pilates? Eat cake?

No, I don't run. I do occasionally do Pilates. And yes—I do eat cake. In fact, I really love cake. I even popped out of one for my ninety-fifth birthday.

After nearly eight decades in medicine, I've treated many patients who were so bent on finding the perfect diet that they made themselves sick; others who were so afraid of dying that they nearly gave up living; and almost all of them hoping I might tell them what to put into their smoothies so they could live forever—or at least an extra few years.

Unfortunately, even after more than a hundred years on this planet, I still have yet to discover a secret ingredient that has been proven to ensure a long and healthy life—well, not one you can put into a blender, anyway.

But I can help you discover the secrets of true health and happiness. They have nothing to do with vitamins or supplements. Instead, they're based on a simple shift in perspective.

Over my many decades in practice, I've come to understand that the point of medicine—and of life—is quite different from what I was taught in medical school. Most people think that the role of medicine is simply to promote physical well-being through putting a stop to whatever ails us. Yet the greater aim is to create a suitably healthy environment—the body—in which the soul can fulfill its purpose.

Each of us came here to do something. And as I see it, true health has nothing to do with diagnosing a disease or prolonging life just for the sake of it; it's about finding out who we are, paying attention to how we're called to grow and change, and listening to what makes our heart sing.

This perspective reflects my larger philosophy: that each individual is part of a greater whole. Just as all the cells in our body work together to sustain life, all living things work together to create the universe we live in. Each of us is therefore both unique and essential.

To understand this broader and more complete view of illness and healing—and of life itself—we need to understand how well-being really works. Contrary to what the medical establishment believes, doctors don't heal patients; only patients can heal themselves. As doctors, we apply skill, knowledge, and ingenuity to treating our patients. We care deeply about people, and we funnel that compassion into our work. This is our sacred role on Earth. Yet ultimately, the best doctors know that healing comes from within.

This may be a surprising admission to hear from a medical doctor like myself. Yet I'm no stranger to alternative views on health. I was born to osteopathic physicians—my mother was one of the first women to graduate with a DO, and my father was both a DO and an MD. They raised me in India, where I was exposed to a wider range of experiences than most of the peers I trained with in medical school. Starting in the 1950s, alongside my husband, Dr. Bill McGarey, I began to research and discuss ideas that were cutting edge at the time: the thought that we are souls having a human experience, that some part of us is interconnected with other people, and that we come here as part of a personal and collective mission of growth and healing. Bill and I were part of the small team that cofounded the American Holistic Medical Association in 1978 with the goal of bringing a holistic understanding—one that unites body, mind, and spirit—to modern Western medicine. I've remained dedicated to that mission ever since.

It's important to note right at the start that holistic medicine is not necessarily what we call alternative medicine; it incorporates a variety of healing modalities, including the allopathic treatments that many know as modern medicine or Western medicine.

The term *holistic medicine* refers not to the strategy but to the approach. It's about treating the whole patient, not just the disease. It's about seeing each individual as a complete and complex being, one with a unique set of physical, psychological, and spiritual characteristics, as well as a personal set of goals to complete in his or her lifetime. The word *holistic* combines *whole* and *holy*, not in a specifically religious sense but in a way that deeply respects the perfection of each human soul and sees the body as an instrument that assists the soul in its tasks. Diseases and symptoms—from simple aches and pains to metastatic cancer—are also part of that perfect design. By showing us where the body is hurt, they show us precisely where the soul needs to work next.

That's why when someone comes in with a headache, I might ask him about his dreams, or when someone comes in with a chronic illness, we might spend our session talking about what happened to her in her childhood. It's the reason many of my patients don't just come to me to discuss only their physical challenges but their emotional and spiritual challenges, too. Each of us is a complex ecosystem of thoughts, feelings, beliefs, and sensations, all of which play into our state of health. I'm not just interested in relieving my patients' symptoms; I'm interested in helping them see their current distress in the context of the greater journey their soul is undertaking.

Life's challenges point us to the part of our soul that is ready to transform. As an acute form of challenge, suffering is a blaring siren that is sure to get our attention. It screams, "Wake up! Pay attention! You have work to do!" Of course, each of us can work to avoid suffering, and we should. But when we approach our own suffering with curiosity, asking it what it may have to teach us, it takes on new meaning. This is true of any kind of suffering—physical, emotional, and spiritual.

When the holistic medical profession says that the mind can influence the body, some people worry that we are saying that the patient caused his or her illness. Others hear that we can learn from our suffering and think that means we deserve it. I understand that people might misinterpret this approach, so I want to clarify: I am not encouraging martyrdom or suggesting that suffering is deserved. I'm also not suggesting that shifting your perspective is the only part of the work. When you have a broken bone, it may need to be reset; when society has a major problem, it may need to be uprooted. Yet even as we work to attend to the physical realities of our bodies and our world, some degree of suffering is unavoidable, so we may as well use it to guide us forward.

This is because although our well-being is *related* to the challenges we face, it isn't entirely *governed* by them. Many people live with diseases and even great pain while remaining joyfully connected to their purpose. Others are disease-free and still wake up not wanting to be alive. Health doesn't require us to live in a problem-free body, just as happiness doesn't require us to experience a problem-free life. Health and happiness are about being so connected to our own life force that we feel we fit into the world around us.

True health is about living *with* the world around us as an engaged, participatory experience. It's about cooperating with the living force within us: our will, our desire to be here and to share our gifts with the world. Our willingness to do so becomes our sense of purpose, and once we have that, our souls can be healthy in any state.

In this book, I will guide you in finding and activating your healing and your learning throughout your life so that you can live each day to the fullest. I will share with you the six profound secrets that can help us in the process that I call *turning toward life*. But you are ultimately in charge of the process. You are the one living your life, and in the end, you are the one who can truly heal it. Your health and vitality—and, yes, your purpose and your happiness, as well—depend on creating a doctor-patient relationship with your own self where you are listening closely to what feeds you and brings you joy, as well as prescribing, for yourself, the healing you most need.

If I could distill my life's work—and my purpose in writing this book—into one sentence, it's this: **To be truly alive, we must find the life force within ourselves and direct our energy toward it.** This shifts our orientation, calling us to face everything in life and engage with it. You may be thinking to yourself: *I engage with my life! After all, I'm the one living it!* But I'm referring to a joyful, participatory engagement that extends to every breath and every moment. I'm talking about dancing a two-step with life itself, finding our willingness and our positivity to keep dancing no matter what it throws our way. When life gets tough, we don't drag our feet; instead, we become curious and we engage even more. Even in the depths of our challenge, we still have access to gratitude.

Along the way, I'll introduce you to some of the incredible patients whom I have had the privilege to support as they connected more deeply with their soul's purpose, embraced joy more fully, and learned how to accept love and care from sometimes unlikely sources. In some cases, their healing was nothing short of miraculous, but there was a science behind those seeming miracles. It involved their aligning with the life energy within themselves.

You'll notice that each of those people had to actively participate in their healing. They had to shift their perspective willingly, using whatever life force they had. I treated them all with love as I helped them face their challenges. Some healed from their physical malady, while others learned to make peace with a chronic condition. Some eventually died, while others lived nearly as long as I have. All got closer to their soul health. They reconnected with their reason for living, and they lived well.

In addition to these stories from my practice, I'll share stories from outside the clinic. My unusual life path has taken me all over the world, and it's been long enough to give me some good stories to tell. I get as much purpose from my role as a mother, grandmother, great-grandmother, and now even great-great-grandmother as I have from my role as a doctor, so I've included bits about that as well. I learn something new every day, and I've had many opportunities to practice what I preach.

I was also blessed to be influenced by a host of extraordinary people. I'll introduce you to my parents, Dr. John Taylor and Dr. Magdelene Elizabeth "Beth" Siehl Taylor, who were pioneering osteopaths and people of faith. They devoted their lives to treating underserved populations in India and raised me and my four siblings there between world wars I and II. You'll meet two of those siblings—my brother Dr. Carl Taylor and my sister, Margaret Taylor Courtwright—both of whom joyfully faced every moment right up until they died. You'll meet my uncompromising Aunt Belle and Harday, our beloved nanny, whom we called "Ayah." (Ayah and her husband, Dar, who cooked for us, were members of our family, though I acknowledge that we would likely call her by a different name today.) You'll also encounter several familiar names of trailblazing public figures whose lives serendipitously intersected with mine.

As you read the stories of my patients and my life, I hope you'll be able to make more sense of your own. It's my intention to help you explore what might be happening to you, so you can understand your own unique body and soul and take charge of your own life and healing. I've treated thousands of patients, and no two were the same. You're forging your own path in life. Your soul is on its own sacred mission, housed in your unique and brilliant body, and only you can direct that process.

Through these stories, you'll connect with my six secrets on a personal level. Much of my philosophy used to be on the edge of accepted truth, but science is catching up! I maintain that it's important for us to embrace science, because it provides us a clear, concrete way of understanding the world. I'm pro-science because I'm pro-question—I like to dig into things and figure them out. At the same time, being pro-question means understanding that there is plenty that science hasn't explained yet. It's always worth asking a question, even if we don't yet know the answer.

I'll also help you ground my six secrets in your heart and body through a series of simple exercises. Each secret includes a small contemplative practice, which I encourage you to do however you see fit—on a walk, with pen and paper, or any other way that calls you. None of these is a cure-all; they're more of what my mother would call "make-dos," which ask us to make the most of what we have been given. And they certainly aren't homework, because I always hated homework! Instead, they are small practices that can inspire a new, holistic perspective on how to live life well.

Hopefully, if you practice them enough times, these exercises can become habits that you can bring into your daily life. You are welcome to adapt them however you need, because if you take one thing from this book, I hope it's that you are absolutely capable of directing your own health and healing as well as your own life and learning. I believe that it isn't enough to just talk about these ideas, we also need to live them—we need to make them real by feeling them in our bodies. So as you're thinking about these topics, I've offered simple ways for you to act them out, feeling into them through embodied practice.

If you've picked up this book, you're already on the journey of aligning with your soul and connecting with your purpose. But none of us can do this alone—especially not right now.

Throughout our lives, many of us find ourselves asking deep, burning questions: *Who am I, truly? Why am I here? How should I spend my days—doing what, and with whom? When this is all over, what is going to have made life worth living?* Faced with uncertainty from all angles, these questions feel even more urgent today.

I want you to access the wisdom deep inside you that enjoys engaging with these questions and isn't in a rush to answer them. I want to help you see what's possible when you connect with your own truth—no matter what anyone else has to say about it.

Before we get started, I have a story to share.

In early 1930, I was onboard a train from Delhi to Bombay (now Mumbai) with my family, feeling sorry for myself to be returning to the United States, where I would be subjected to ironed dresses and proper manners and other things my wild-hearted being just couldn't bear. I'd finally had a teacher I liked at school and was devastated to leave, but my parents assured me that we'd be back soon enough. They had been granted a furlough, and we were going to stay near my father's family wheat farm in Kansas. Little did I know that when we were there, the Great Depression would begin, grounding us in Kansas for more than two years—at nine, I could not comprehend such things. All I knew was that we were leaving India, saying good-bye to Ayah and Dar, and going to a faraway land I had visited only once and didn't remember.

My dusty face was pressed against the bars of the window, watching the beloved land of my birth go by, when the train started to slow. A crowd had gathered along the railroad tracks, following a procession ahead. The women were dressed in their best clothes, and children were dancing and throwing flowers. Up ahead, in the first-class part of the train, everyone continued to sit primly as if nothing were happening. But in the third-class car, where we were sitting, people were climbing out of the windows and running to join the crowd; others ran along the tops of the train cars, their feet thundering on the metal roof.

As the train inched forward and overtook the procession, the people marching ahead began to come into view. In front, there was a small man wearing a simple white *dhoti*—a cloth wrapped around his waist and thighs—and carrying a *larthi*, a wooden staff. Though the sun beat down on him, he sauntered along with joy, fully engaged in his life and purpose. By then people had begun to shout his name, but I already knew I was seeing the legend my parents had told me about with such respect, the man who was lifting the people out of their oppression and into the light of empowerment: *Gandhiji.*

The train stopped, and after hours of feeling its monotonous rumble through my body, the sudden stillness felt electric.

Just then, a child ran up to the mahatma holding a flower. Gandhi stopped, bent down, and received it. As he did, I saw love emanating from his whole being. He stood up to continue marching and looked back over the crowd, viewing not only the people on the ground and rooftops but those of us with our faces pressed against the window bars. And I swear that for a second, he looked directly at me.

I have known love in my life many times over. But the love of that man will never leave me. It felt as if he saw my sadness at leaving India, my fear, my hope, and accepted all of it. He looked at me with an unforgettable love—one that recognized my very soul.

He turned and led the march away.

I was witnessing Gandhi's historic Salt March, or Salt Satyagraha, in which he led a nonviolent protest against the British heavily taxing salt.

If I could give you one thing right now, it would be that same unforgettable love, the kind that recognizes and accepts everything that you are. That love carries the hope for the future. It carries the meaning of many lessons, giving purpose to impossible struggle, signaling the turning point when the force of life swells up and pushes us into a new paradigm.

Whoever you are reading this, please know that I have profound respect for what you came here to do. I hold delicately everything you have been through, and I feel deeply hopeful for what is to come. I can guide you with my six secrets and offer you all the love in the world.

The rest is up to you.

SECRET I

You Are Here
for a Reason

Chapter 1

THE JUICE

I remember the exact moment I first found my juice.

My parents were missionaries near Mussoorie, India, midway up in the Himalayas. From the age of five onward, I was sent with my older siblings to the only English-speaking school in the region, which largely served the children of missionaries, government officials, and officers of the British army. I was a bit of a grubby kid—my mother and my nanny, Ayah, did their best to make sure I was clean and dressed properly, but I did my best to undo their work. I preferred playing in the dirt and climbing trees to playing with dolls or reading books. I liked listening to stories, but I didn't like reading them—every time I looked at the letters, they would swim around on the page, so I couldn't really ever understand what the printed words meant.

At the time, we didn't have a word for this challenge. Today it's called dyslexia. But I spent my early years in school thinking that I was stupid, an idea that was promoted by my first-grade teacher, who would often single me out for my mistakes. I did so poorly in her class that I had to take it twice, and her opinion of me left a deep impression on my sense of self-worth.

Looking back, my struggle seems quite sweet. The fact that I went on to have the career I have had makes it clear in hindsight that it was just a short chapter in my young life. But at the time I struggled mightily. I truly believed I was stupid. I mean, sure, I thought that teacher was even stupider than I was, but I really worried about how I'd be able to make it in the world if I couldn't learn such a simple thing as how to read. Most of all, I worried about my ability to follow my parents into practicing medicine, which was my greatest dream.

I also had an awful time making friends. I was terribly lonely and would count the steps as I walked up the hill home every day after school, waiting until I could curl up under Ayah's shawl to cry.

I spent those two long first-grade years waiting for the winter, when we would all pack up into our caravan and go off into the plains to work. I loved nothing more than the time spent in the mobile camps where my parents treated patients. Ours was a bustling traveling community, to which people from all over the countryside—most of them from the lowest castes of India's oppressive system—would come to receive medical care. The caste system had labeled them "untouchable," which my parents found both inaccurate and tragic. I never understood it either—how could Ayah be "untouchable," when a hug from her was the most wonderful thing in the world? How could Dar, or anyone else, be untouchable, for that matter—anyone at all? My parents also worked with people with leprosy, known today as Hansen's disease, and with women, who often couldn't receive care elsewhere. Most of the people they treated had never seen a doctor before, and very few of them had any money.

That commitment made our camp a busy hub to which people could come not only to receive treatment but to receive love, kindness, and community. We would work from dawn until the hottest hours of the day, rest, and then work again until nightfall. Then we would all sit around the campfire together, telling stories under a blanket of stars.

It seemed that everyone in the area knew when we were around, and they knew my parents would take on any patient who needed help. One day my father took my older brothers hunting, which meant it was up to me, Margaret, and our younger brother, Gordon, to help our mother in the medicine tent. I loved assisting her, helping people with infected wounds, chronic illness, and broken bones. I was proud of the fact that my mother was a doctor. I also felt that I had already seen almost everything in my first eight years of life. But that day, we got a patient we never expected.

Around midday, a commotion began. Then a young man walked into the camp leading a wounded elephant! My mother went to greet him and tried to explain that she was not a veterinarian. But the man told her that he was a very special elephant, the rajah's favorite to ride on a hunt. Some time before, the elephant had stepped on a bamboo stump and injured its foot. The wound simply would not heal. Though the rajah normally had his animals treated by the caretakers, he knew my parents were in the area, and he had instructed the man, who was the elephant's trainer, not to return until they had treated the elephant personally.

My mother had never worked with an elephant before, yet she was not one to shy away from a challenge. With a gentle yet confident tone, she started by talking to the elephant as she would to any other nervous patient. "Let's have a look here," she said in a soothing voice. "I'll be gentle. I can see it hurts a good deal." She looked carefully at the elephant's left front foot, gingerly touching the tender pad. It was in fact quite infected, and she deduced that a splinter of the bamboo must still be inside. It was exciting but slightly intimidating to be close to such a majestic animal. I was surprised by his gentle energy as I ran my hand along his wrinkled skin and smooth tusks.

Sensing my desire to help, my mother sent me to get forceps, potassium permanganate, and a large copper syringe. I first brought the forceps and the biggest syringe we had in our set of supplies. My mother was still speaking in her soothing tone—"There, there, you're doing a wonderful job"—as the elephant stood, patient and blinking.

I then went back into the medical tent to prepare the antiseptic solution. I got a large bottle of potassium permanganate down from a shelf—our medical tent was always meticulously organized—and put it beside the jug of water we kept there. Then I measured out the solution carefully, filling an entire basin with the purple liquid while avoiding contact with the strong chemical, which I knew would scald my skin if undiluted. I lifted the heavy, wide basin in my hands and slowly walked back outside, taking care to not slosh the liquid onto the uneven ground below. When I returned, I found the elephant standing quietly as he watched my mother probe for the bamboo wood lodged deep in the smooth gray pad of his front foot. He patiently allowed her to remove the long splinter and irrigate the infection underneath. I could understand why the rajah loved that elephant so much. He was so well mannered that he didn't even flinch.

When she had finished cleaning the wound, my mother smeared an ointment on it to complete the treatment. Elephants are expressive animals, and that one seemed pleased—so pleased, in fact, that when it was time for the man to take him over to the Ganges River to cool off, the elephant reached down with his trunk to lift Margaret, who squealed with delight and fear, right up into the air. We held our breath. But he proceeded to plop her down onto his back, and we exhaled with relief. Then he reached down for me.

Seeing what had happened to Margaret, I wasn't afraid. I relished the leathery curve that snaked around me, feeling the powerful muscle that made his nose so wildly different from my own. I had seen many elephants before and watched them feed themselves from trees and lift their young—but I had never touched one of their impressive trunks or imagined what it would feel like to have one squeeze around me. I didn't have long to ponder that, though, because in short order I found myself sitting beside my sister, the elephant's back wide beneath me. Then he reached down for our brother Gordon, who put his small hands around my waist when he arrived behind me. And off we went! We rode down to the river as the other camp children followed, and when we arrived, the elephant playfully sprayed us all. Though the water was usually off limits due to the snakes and crocodiles, the adults knew that none would come near us with the elephant there, so we stayed and played with him all afternoon.

The next day, the man brought the elephant back to camp so my mother could check the wound for signs of infection. The elephant went straight to her and wrapped his trunk around her waist, lifting her up into the air as he had me and my siblings. For the rest of the week, the elephant visited every day and, as if to demonstrate his gratitude, greeted my mother with a big trunk hug, to which she responded with her usual humor, laughing as she joyfully called out, "Now, be a good boy and put me down!" Afterward, we would all go to the river to play, sometimes riding the elephant through the shallows, other times screaming as he showered us with water from his trunk.

It was a pivotal time in my life. When I started school the following year, I was pleased to find that I didn't hate it so much after all.

Helping my mother treat the elephant helped me discover that I was born to be a doctor. Though dyslexia always made school hard for me, I learned that it has no bearing on my intelligence. My new teacher understood my dilemma and found a way to teach me to read, and knowing that I would need to be able to as a medical student gave me the courage to follow her direction. I began to believe in myself again. That understanding brought me the rest of the way through school, then college, and then medical school.

Like my parents, healing gave me an opportunity to interact with the world in a positive and meaningful way. When I was carrying the purple solution out to that elephant, I connected so deeply with my joy that I realized my school troubles wouldn't stop me—I'd find a way to make it through. I knew I was important and needed. I felt I was a part of things.

We all deserve to feel this way. Each of us is here for a reason, to learn and grow and to give our gifts. When we are able to do so, we're filled with the creative life energy that I call the "juice."

The juice is our reason for living. It's our fulfillment, our joy. It's what happens when life is activated by love. It's the energy we get from the things that matter and mean something to us. It's what my parents got from their work with underserved populations, and it's the first secret I share with you: *You are here for a reason.* **Each of us is here to connect with our unique gifts; this is what activates our desire to be alive.** Achieving this connection isn't necessarily the point. The search counts for far more.

The process of "finding our juice" keeps us vital.

This concept isn't new—nor is the idea that it's related to health. Numerous Eastern philosophies have noted that there is a certain energy tied to well-being; it's been called both *prana* and *chi*. Western philosophers may refer to something more theoretical, such as motivation or purpose. Emergency medical workers and hospice care professionals often describe juice as a will to live, because when a person loses it, he or she starts to die. Though being juiced doesn't ensure perfect health, running out or losing our juice is often a major obstacle to feeling good.

We're all called to find our juice through our daily contribution to the world. Certain activities and pursuits bring us more juice, and this varies from person to person. Some people find a vocation that lights them up, and they spend their whole careers pinching themselves and thinking "I can't believe I'm getting paid for this!" Others work less juicy jobs to make a living and pursue their passions off the clock. Still others, such as unpaid caregivers, contribute to society in other important ways while still connecting with their unique sense of purpose.

Though there is no one way or one area of life to find our juice, we all need to find it; it's a vital part of our life force. Without juice, it's hard to feel joy, and both physical and mental health start to waver. This is part of why I often find myself asking patients what they have to live *for*, because if they can't answer this question, I can often only relieve their symptoms temporarily. I may fix what's wrong, but I can't necessarily make it right.

If we're lucky, we've experienced juice plenty of times in our lives. Yet just as often, many of us find our juice seems to run out. This can be a shocking and notable experience. But it can also be much subtler, like a car that putters, sputters, and runs out of gas.

Chapter 2

WHY AM I HERE?

Not everyone finds their path as young as I did. Many struggle to find out who they really are and what gives them juice. It can be something that lives inside us right under the surface, but feels just beyond our reach. That was the case for James.

James was a recent computer science graduate who was not sure what to do next. I had treated him and his parents for many years. He had come to see me at his mother's urging, but after a quick history and physical it was clear that there was nothing wrong—at least with his body. He had a Walkman clipped to his jeans—yes, it was that long ago—and wore the headphones around his neck as his eyes darted around the room nervously.

"What is worrying you, James?"

"I just don't know what to do with my life. I have this degree and student loans to pay, but I'm just not interested in any of the job listings."

"Do you like computers?"

"Not really, but I know computers are a big thing. My father is an engineer, and he thinks it's a safe career. The way the world is going, I'm not sure any place is safe."

"What do you want to do?"

"I don't know," he said, but I suspected that some part of his unconscious mind might. It just wasn't safe for him to admit it, even to himself.

"Have you had any dreams?"

He told me that he occasionally dreamed about a tall cactus but didn't remember anything else, so I suggested we do a visualization, and he agreed. I said, "Close your eyes and look around you. Can you see a path? It could be cobblestones, a dirt trail, a paved road, even a sidewalk."

Jim furrowed his brow, then his forehead went slack. "There," he whispered.

"Start to walk down the path. Take one step, and then another and another," I said. "Now look around. This is your path. What do you see on it?"

"I'm up on the mesa," Jim said quietly after a minute.

"Look way up ahead. What do you see there?"

Jim's brow furrowed again. "I see that cactus. I hear some drumming. I don't know." He opened his eyes. "Dr. Gladys, I just don't know. There's so much I need to figure out. I asked my parents if I could go up to the mesa and camp by myself, but they are nervous. They want to know if I'm on drugs. I just want to be alone and connect with nature."

"I think you should go. If your parents have a problem, have them call me."

I saw James at the supermarket several weeks later, and he told me he had gone up onto the mesa by himself. He said it had been a vision quest. He told me he had heard drumming in his head the whole time he was there and that he knew what he wanted to do. He wanted to become a musician, and he was going to enroll in graduate school for music production. I could see the light sparkling in his eyes. He was filled with juice.

"What do your parents think?"

"They are worried about me being a starving musician with my debt, but they've agreed for me to try it for a year and see if I can make it in music."

As James's story shows, sometimes finding our juice pushes us to go through a transition in life. It shows us who we really are. This may require us to make a change, start doing something new, or stop doing something we've done for quite some time.

In other cases, very little external shift is needed.

Lilian had everything and nothing at the same time. She was sitting right there next to me, but her mind seemed far away when she said, "There's just something wrong with me, I'm sure of it."

I'd been her doctor for many years and had also treated other members of her family, and they generally seemed like a happy bunch. Her grown children were polite and successful. Her marriage was secure. She was well connected in the community and enjoyed volunteering for a local nonprofit serving low-income children.

Though Lilian had presented various symptoms in the past, all of which had been resolved, her current complaints were vague. Maybe she was sick, she suggested, or there was a tumor we didn't know about. She thought perhaps she was in the early stages of an autoimmune disorder or her hormones were out of balance. She was unwell, she was just sure of it, and she trusted me to help her figure it out.

I began by asking Lilian about her symptoms more specifically. Did her head hurt? No. How about her digestion? Fine, regular, no problems. Was any part of her body in pain? Not really; she felt herself aging, so she occasionally noticed a little twinge here or there, but nothing in particular. I probed for psychological symptoms next, asking if she was sleeping well (yes) and whether she had been experiencing panic attacks or depression (no). But she just felt . . . *bad.* "I just don't have energy for anything anymore," she explained. "I've been put in charge of the annual fundraiser for the children's society, but I can hardly complete the work—it just feels like I'm going through the motions."

Lilian isn't the only patient to share this kind of experience—they can't quite describe the exact symptoms, which sometimes shift every day. Some weeks it's aches and pains that seem to affect everything. Sometimes they just seem devoid of energy. Sometimes they just feel unengaged. Lilian couldn't name any of that, but she seemed to be suffering from all three.

Finally I asked her what was really going on. "Lilian," I said gently, "what do *you* think is wrong?"

She looked down at her soft, manicured hands. It took her a minute to answer, and I could tell that she was searching deep inside herself to name something she had not yet been able to define. In those long seconds, we waited together.

Then she said it. "I guess I don't have anything to live for anymore."

Her words hung thick in the air as we both breathed in their gravity.

After a few seconds, Lilian cut through the silence, attempting to explain. "I mean, I have everything in my life I've always wanted," she said. "I like my life. I have nothing to complain about. But—" She faltered and gazed around the room, touching the delicate necklace she wore at her throat as though trying to put her finger on the nature of her dissatisfaction.

"Nobody needs me anymore. I don't feel like my life has any meaning," she said at last. Her voice shook and the tears began to roll down her cheeks. "My boys don't live at home anymore. My husband has his work, and it doesn't seem to really matter what I do for these children because their problems never really go away. It's more depressing than anything else. What am I even here for? I've already done everything I needed to do, and there's no point in being alive." Lilian began tugging more urgently at her necklace, her anxiety mounting. "I don't know what to do next. Maybe there *is* nothing to do next. Maybe I'm done."

Even when it seems as though we have everything, we have nothing without juice. Living without juice is an emptiness, a listlessness. It's not quite clinical depression, but it's not quite being alive, either. As Lilian described it, it just *feels bad*.

This book includes many remarkable stories of people dramatically turning toward life. But Lilian's story has always remained close to my heart because most of life isn't that dramatic. It's more often day by day, minute by minute, either engaging with the world around us or . . . not. Many of the most pivotal shifts happen in patients like this one.

I pulled Lilian in and hugged her fiercely, silently commending her bravery. No one ever taught me to hug people in medical school—today, they probably teach people *not* to—but I've always done it anyway.

Then I tried to explain to her what was happening.

"You matter, Lilian. You've just forgotten," I said. "You're part of something bigger than yourself. You're part of your son's lives, your husband's life, your friends' lives. You are a part of life itself. You aren't done. Your life isn't over. It's right there, waiting for you to engage with it." I told her how in my mind's eye, I saw Lilian and saw her life. It was as if I could draw two circles around them that did not touch. They were separate. How could her life give her juice like that? And how could she give anything back in return?

We discussed her role in the community a little more, and she seemed to lighten just a bit. Intellectually, she seemed to understand what I was telling her. But her body hadn't caught up yet.

A few days later, Lilian had a fall. She was stepping off her patio when her ankle twisted and she hit the pavement, shattering her right hip.

I heard about her fall and went to visit her in the hospital. It had already been almost two weeks since the accident, and she was very depressed. She brightened when she saw me, but then her sorrow returned.

"How are you spending your time in here, Lilian?" I asked after I gave her a big, long hug.

"I'm doing nothing at all. I can't do anything. I have to stay here in bed," she answered.

"Well, your arms work. Your mind works. Surely you can do something, and you must, because if you stay here like this you'll run out of juice entirely."

Lilian looked at me strangely. "What can I do from a hospital bed?" she asked.

"Well, who is planning the fundraiser for the children's society?" I asked.

She explained that in her absence, an employee of the nonprofit had been put in charge of the fundraiser, but in truth he was too overworked to really do anything. I encouraged her to call up the employee and ask to take some of the responsibilities back. "You have to reconnect with your life force, and for that to happen, you have to get busy," I counseled her. "Your hip needs to heal, but if you stay down in the dumps it's going to take a lot longer."

Lilian took what I said to heart. She started planning the event from her hospital bed. She became energized by choosing decorations, arranging speakers, and deciding on a menu. Two months later, I went to her fundraiser—and it was one of the most beautiful events I'd ever attended. The money she helped raise started a whole new after-school program for children in need.

Both Lilian and James were at my 102nd birthday this year. It was wonderful having them celebrate with me, and I got to celebrate the juice-filled lives that they've created. Lilian still works with the children's society, leading the annual fundraiser. Decades after his first trip up the mountain, James became a respected brother in the local Native American tribe and leads others on vision quests, which supplements his career as a highly successful professional musician.

Watching them both thrive reminded me that our search for juice connects us to the greater question of *why we're here*. Some of us are spiritually inclined, some identify as religious, and others place their respect in the perfect randomness of the universe. But regardless of the *how* behind our understanding of creation, our juice speaks to the *why*. Juice is the immediate result of our reaching for life and its reaching back to us.

It's important that we be the ones to initiate this movement, but once we do, the juice that starts flowing stays flowing. It expands until we are so filled with juice that we begin to connect with something even greater: purpose.

That's right: lives filled with juice become lives filled with purpose. And that has a profound effect not only on our mental health but on our physical health, too. Several analyses of the University of Michigan Health and Retirement Study have observed a link between a high sense of purpose and decreased mortality in adults over fifty.[1] Purpose has been found to reduce the risk of cardiovascular events[2] and to prevent the worst effects of Alzheimer's disease.[3] There is also evidence linking volunteerism with decreased risk of death—not to mention a stronger sense of well-being.[4] This suggests that living with purpose can actually help us live longer—and better.

And the joy it brings to our lives will ripple out to the world around us. In holistic medicine, we don't just understand the body's well-being as an aspect of the soul's well-being—we consider a soul's well-being as an aspect of the world's well-being. We improve the health of the world when we tend to our souls and our hearts, because we all fit together.

Chapter 3

LIKE PIECES OF A
JIGSAW PUZZLE

My mother might never have ended up in medical school had it not been for Mrs. Gimble, the grumpy old neighbor who lived three doors down. She walked with a pronounced limp and complained nearly constantly of pain in her spine that the doctors couldn't heal. But one day in 1910 when my mother was on the porch, Mrs. Gimble came striding evenly down the street and smiling.

Could it really be the same woman?

What was the reason for her complete change in demeanor?

Mrs. Gimble told my mother she had been treated by an osteopathic doctor who had twisted her around like a pretzel on the dining room table, healing her pain once and for all. Dr. Andrew Still, the founder of osteopathic medicine, was very progressive—so progressive, Mrs. Gimble proclaimed, that he had even started accepting women into his medical school.

My mother had never heard of an osteopathic doctor, but she wanted to make grumpy people smile again. She was thrilled by the idea that she could train to do so under Dr. Still. She got to work finding out what she needed to do to apply.

Within the year she'd joined one of the first coed cohorts. There she met my father and graduated in 1913. She spent the rest of her life bringing healing to people in pain. My parents treated countless patients at the women's hospital they started in Rourkee, India; in the field camps they ran every winter; and in the small Kansas community where we lived during the Great Depression. In most cases, they took little or no money for their work. Beyond her role as a healer, my mother was an inspiration to many, as thousands of people were exposed to her as the first woman doctor they ever knew.

Mrs. Gimble changed my mother's life by helping her connect to her purpose, and my mother went on to change many lives through her healing work in India and beyond. This is precisely how juice works—it not only connects us to our own purpose but binds us together through collective purpose.

By collective purpose, I don't mean that we all have the *same* purpose. Rather, I mean that when we're juiced, we contribute to the greater sense of purpose that ripples out from those with whom we interact to our greater community. Our individual souls are like pieces of a jigsaw puzzle. Our purpose locks us together, creating something greater and more beautiful than any of us could achieve alone.

I like thinking of us as puzzle pieces because it gives us each space to be unique. We're not supposed to be shaped this way or that; we're supposed to be shaped precisely as we are, because that way we can fit together. It isn't anyone's job to judge the shape of anyone else's piece, and in the same way, it isn't useful to try to make ourselves more or less like anyone else or to worry if they judge our shape. Instead, it's up to each of us to align with our own soul and help others do the same. Seeing things this way helps us understand that each of us is essential. Have you ever nearly finished a jigsaw puzzle only to find that there's a piece missing? It's a crisis!

When we don't find our place in the puzzle, we feel a bit lumpy and misshapen. We might wonder why we are the way we are. We might compare ourselves to others or feel that we aren't beautiful enough on our own. We don't see ourselves in the larger whole, which can make us feel hopeless, depressed, and isolated. We feel small and insignificant, as though we have no power over our lives and no reason for existing.

But when we feel ourselves click into the whole puzzle, we become part of the pattern of life. When this happens, we exchange juice with the world around us. Our juice flows freely, and we have more of it than ever before.

Each of us spends our lifetime discovering the shape of our own puzzle piece.

When I went to medical school a generation after my mother, there were only a few schools that accepted women into their ranks. I attended Woman's Medical College of Pennsylvania in Philadelphia, the only all-women's school, where we were told that we would have to be smarter, tougher, and overall better doctors to survive. My cohort started just as World War II began.

I had come because I wanted to love and heal people. But it seemed to me that the country's focus on war had bled into the medical establishment—or maybe it had always been that way and I hadn't noticed before. I followed what my parents had done, treating physical health as a single part of a larger ecosystem. I was less focused on killing a disease and more interested in why it was there. That put me at odds with the education I was receiving. Though I could follow the anatomy, biology, and other hard science, I struggled with the whole approach to diagnosis and treatment that I was being offered in school.

That, combined with my tendency to knit while in class to keep my busy mind focused, made me the least favorite of the dean, stiff old Marion Fay. Dean Fay thought about as much of me as my first-grade teacher had, and she made her opinion known.

One day she pulled me into her office, where I'd been lectured and belittled many times before. She sat perfectly upright, glasses hanging on a chain over her crisp white blouse, not a bit of softness to be seen. "Miss Taylor, I have a referral here for a psychiatrist."

"A psychiatrist?" I laughed incredulously.

"I'm not sure if you're *quite right*," she continued, tapping a pencil against her temple as she said the last two words to indicate her meaning. "You don't seem to understand the point of medicine at all. You spend all day just knitting during class. Perhaps you weren't cut out to be a doctor. The psychiatrist will ascertain if that is so."

"Respectfully, ma'am, aren't we meant to participate in our own education?" I asked. "We're the ones who will be sent out to hospitals and clinics when this is all over. Isn't it imperative that we truly understand the concepts behind the teachings? Everything here is about killing—we're never talking about how love can heal."

"It's *your* concepts that worry me," she said, gripping her pencil tightly. "Medicine *is* about killing disease, because it's disease that kills people and it's our job to keep them alive. What is this all about love and healing? You're so soft you're almost like a nurse. You need to be tough, Miss Taylor. You'll never make it through residency like that."

I set my mouth in a line to keep it from running, managed a tight "Thank you," and rushed out of the room as quickly as I could, grasping that horrible referral paper in my hand.

I did go to the psychiatrist—and he deemed me right as rain. But the experience shook me to my core. I understood that the medical establishment was never going to accept me as I was. Looking back, that was the moment I realized I would have to make my mark on medicine by doing things my own way.

If I'd let them, those four years in medical school could have sapped the juice right out of me. I kept focused on the goal: I just had to make it through. Once I was a doctor, I could focus on love and healing, even if I had to focus on killing disease to get there. This idea gave me juice—as did the letters I exchanged with my beau, Bill McGarey, who was attending medical school in Cincinnati.

I kept on studying, graduated, and received the title of medical doctor. I had earned my place in the medical community. I married Bill in 1943, and shortly after we both graduated, we went into private practice together.

My understanding of healing evolved through the years, and I came to believe in the concept of reincarnation, which was greatly at odds with the theology I'd been taught as a child. With Bill at my side, I started pushing myself beyond the boundaries of everything I was taught to believe. I came to understand that the scientific community is not in full agreement about what consciousness is, and where it comes from. That helped me embrace the idea that our spirits are ageless and are meant to learn over multiple lifetimes. Bill and I emerged at the center of a growing movement of physicians and healers who were interested in the spiritual and soulful aspects of medicine, and today, a belief in reincarnation guides much of what I do on Earth as a doctor, mother, grandmother, and human being. It reinforces my conviction that each of us comes here for a purpose—and that each of our individual purposes is connected, as our souls interact with other souls over the course of many lifetimes.

It also helped me click into the world around me. Many years later the shape of my own puzzle piece developed more clearly, and I was able to connect ever more closely with my juice. I came to understand much more about what I am here to do—not only to be a medical doctor and mother but to promote both new and ancient ideas about healing on the *soul* level, not only the physical. It furthered my understanding of the type of medicine my parents had promoted and solidified my disagreement with the modern medical establishment's focus on killing. As I came to see it, our health challenges are as much a part of our soul's journey as anything else is. Our goal should not be simply to kill them off but to allow them to help us grow and learn at the same time.

Exploring the intersection of spirituality and medicine is a significant part of my role. But what if we don't know what our role is or how to follow it as it changes? And what happens when we feel called to so many things that we're pulled in several directions?

Chapter 4

WHERE SHOULD I POUR
MY JUICE?

Not long ago I met a young woman named Anne who was dealing with her third major bout of bronchitis in less than a year. She came into my office with a barking cough that sounded painful. I began with questions about her lifestyle: Did she smoke or work in a place with poor ventilation? No, that wasn't it. Then I asked her a bit about her medical history: any allergies or respiratory illnesses?

"No," she said, her voice hoarse. "Not really."

"Are you using your voice a lot?"

"That depends," she said with a laugh, which quickly turned into coughing. Between sputters she joked, "Is twenty-four hours a day too much?"

She told me that she loved her job in film production, but there were so many meetings that her voice was usually gone by Wednesday. When she left the office, she headed straight to a yoga studio to pursue her other passion: teaching yoga four nights a week.

As she spoke about her two jobs, it was clear that they lit her up. But she knew she had to slow down. If she was really honest with herself, she no longer loved teaching yoga the way she once had, but she'd invested so much time and energy into it that to walk away would feel like failure. Worse, she feared that she would lose her identity if she didn't pursue yoga as part of her career. Yet she admitted that it was exhausting to teach as much as she did, and it created a chaotic schedule in which she had trouble giving her body the care it needed.

Shortly after our conversation, Anne cut back teaching yoga to just once a week. She still went to the studio most evenings, but she started taking classes instead of teaching them. When she came back a month later, I could already see that things were much better. Her voice was clear, and she was barely coughing at all. I listened to her lungs, and it sounded as though she was on the mend.

"How are you feeling about your new schedule?" I asked.

"It's funny—I thought I would miss teaching, but it is so much more relaxing just to be a student. I've started going to the later class, which is a slower, gentler practice than the early-evening class I taught. It gives me time for a light dinner in my own kitchen that I have time to digest—before, I was grabbing meals on the go late at night and falling asleep full." She told me that she was coughing less and felt herself better able to breathe. "I guess it's a little strange, like I've moved backward in my spiritual practice, though."

I was puzzled. "Why would that represent moving *backward* in your spiritual practice?"

"Well, I was a successful yoga teacher before, and now I'm mostly a student."

I smiled. Her response was so lovely—and so misguided. "Anne, you're finally living what you're teaching," I explained. "It's not degrees or labels that help you understand what's going on inside of you. It's not a job that tells you whether you're spiritual or not."

Anne gave a small laugh, acknowledging what I'd said.

"Some of the wisest people I've ever known are barbers or kitchen workers," I went on, thinking of Ayah, who never learned to read and write. "You were stretching beyond where your heart wanted to go, and your body was trying to tell you that. Thank it. It showed you exactly what you needed to see."

"That makes sense," Anne said, speaking slowly as she mulled over the thought. "I guess it looks like I have less going on from the outside, but I feel much better now that I'm not trying to do it all." In the months that followed, she continued to improve. By giving up on spreading herself too thin, she could take better care of her health and well-being.

In today's busy culture, it can be hard to find our own right way. We often want to be successful in everything we do, and we're encouraged to judge our success from the outside—whether we're good at doing something or whether it makes us money or brings us prestige. But in truth, happiness has much more to do with how we feel than anything else. When we try to follow everyone else, do what we think we "should," or create an identity for ourselves that doesn't work, we suffer.

Many people learn this the hard way through the experience of parenthood. Some people love being parents, while others are drained by it.

For me, motherhood was always a source of juice. I always dreamed of having six children, and Bill and I agreed upon the number before we were even married. I worked outside the home during a time when it wasn't common for women to do so. I was well into medical school when the Rosie the Riveter image made its debut. Because I was working and had four children in four years, I was often questioned about my family planning. "You would think that *you*, of all people, would know how to stop having babies," a bitter patient snapped at me one day. She was frustrated that she was being treated by a woman doctor and, due to her prejudice, probably a little bit afraid that I wouldn't do a good job. By that time, I was juggling raising my kids while running a busy medical practice as one of the only general practitioners in town. I remember my shock at her statement—she couldn't imagine that perhaps I'd chosen to have all four children or that I'd go on to joyfully have two more. But I did, and I always found kind women in the neighborhood—usually a generation above me and often lacking some juice themselves after their own children had left the house—whom I hired to stay home with the children while I worked.

Having two distinct sources of juice always seemed to tug me in two directions. At work, I worried about what was happening at home; at home, I worried about my patients.

Many people have similar concerns. To be interested and engaged in life often brings this sense of being tugged in multiple directions toward different passions, each of which requires time, attention, and life force. Where should we pour our juice? It feels as though we have to make a choice, but we're complex beings, and we're meant to embrace that complexity. From what I've seen, the happiest people juggle multiple interests. My son John is a pastor who always felt inclined toward technology, so he enjoys setting up equipment for church presentations as well as my interviews and video calls. His namesake, my brother John, was a minister, hunter, and dentist who returned to India after his formal retirement to pull teeth and treat abscesses. A dear friend of mine today is a professional writer but enjoys working with horses, growing vegetables, and singing in the church choir. All of them found a way to make enough money with one of their passions to support the others, which has led to fulfilling, well-rounded lives.

In my case, I found that my roles as mother and physician somehow supported each other. It was a different time, when child care wasn't inexpensive but didn't break the bank, either. At the time, plenty of people suggested that I was less of a mother because I worked, and plenty of male doctors (and even female nurses!) seemed to think I was less of a doctor because I had so many kids. I just kept on doing what was true to me, getting juice from work and home equally. Coming home to my children's warm smiles gave me juice to go back to the office the next morning, and interacting with my patients renewed my juice to continue giving the kids all I had. Later, as my career expanded to speaking, writing, and bringing new ideas to people, I saw that instead of running out of juice, I seemed to get more and more of it.

As with parenting, we can get juice from gardening, sports, out-door pursuits, activism, artistry, or any number of other activities, even if they aren't our official "jobs." In my generation, people had plenty of hobbies. Entertainment was an event that often took place outside the home, so we had to come up with ways to entertain ourselves. Many of us cooked from scratch, worked on our homes and cars, gardened, wrote stories, sang and played musical instruments, or practiced crafts such as knitting, cross-stitching, and painting. Such activities are cre-ative and connect us with our life force. It didn't matter much whether we were good or bad at what we did—the point was simply to enjoy doing it.

I've noticed that through the decades, people have become less interested in such activities. Constant access to entertainment and devices makes it hard to pursue things that are challenging. With the pressures of modern life, it's often hard to see the value in pursuits that don't make money or immediately solve widespread problems. It's hard for many people to understand why they should do things just for the sake of doing them. I was heartened to see that during the Covid pandemic, younger generations began to pick up such ac-tivities again.

Young people—and by that I mean anyone under ninety-nine, but especially those in their teens and twenties—need such activities to help release stress, because today's world is exposing us to every crisis that has ever occurred in real time. We're more aware than ever of societal imbalance, a lack of social justice, and the current and impending consequences of the way we're treating our planet. Seen from one angle, this is incredibly useful information; seen from another, it's useful only if we use it. And if we don't, if we allow it to freeze us up and cut us off from doing anything that could bring us joy, we will lose touch with our own life force, making it even less likely that we'll be able to do anything to help.

We're able to connect with life best when we get juice from mul-tiple places. A puzzle piece doesn't just click in on one side; it clicks in on two, three, or four. What that looks like varies from person to person. As Anne at the beginning of this chapter learned, sometimes backing off from the things we love can shake our sense of identity, but it's sometimes the only way to bring ourselves back to balance. As we learn and grow, we come to realize that our juice has nothing to do with external definitions and everything to do with how we show up for our lives in the day-to-day.

Anne's story also shows us that our sources of juice are meant to change over time. Usually, this experience feels natural. We enjoy something for a while, then find something that catches our interest even more and move on. Life twists and turns, our interests change, and our physical abilities shift as we age.

When life is truly flowing, what gives us juice evolves alongside us. Sometimes our struggle to get juice is exactly the thing that pushes us to find it somewhere else, such as a master electrician who was devastated when a disability forced him into early retirement, only to discover the restorative powers of gardening, or a film producer who threw herself fully into volunteering at a local shelter during the early days of the Covid pandemic. At the time, they thought that what was happening was a disaster, but when they look back on their lives, they see that life itself was calling them to keep looking for their juice and that it was the second pursuit that kept them alive. The very fact that they were determined to find their juice—the inner calling, the desire within them—was how they reconnected with life.

Chapter 5

CONNECTING WITH DESIRE

Living with juice calls upon us to name what we want. But when we first start turning toward life, it can be scary to even *know* what we want, let alone speak it aloud.

We tell ourselves that maybe we want too much. We may think that we shouldn't want anything at all. Or we can't seem to decide exactly what we want, and even when we do, we may think that it's silly or unattainable. We may even be so hurt and confused that we convince ourselves that we don't want anything at all.

If you can relate, take a minute to close your eyes. Just for a moment, let yourself want. Let yourself yearn for whatever it is you wish for yourself and your life: the conversation you're afraid to have, the job you thought you'd never be good enough to do, the friendships and laughter you miss from another time in your life, or even a really good bar of chocolate.

Just *want.*

This is life moving through you. Life wants—it calls, it yearns, it desires. We have to first accept that this is true. Only then can our hearts whisper to us what they want most of all.

I think back to that young version of me—the one who couldn't read and who was bullied on the playground. On a small scale, I wanted specific things. I wanted a new teacher, a new set of eyes that could read, and just one school friend to confide in. Yet I wanted something much greater, too: I wanted to be able to serve. I wanted to know that my struggles in school weren't going to hold me back my whole life. I wanted to know that even though things were very hard, they were going to get better somehow.

As I explained in chapter 1, every day I would walk home from school to our bungalow on the mountainside. The road was steep and about a mile long. Way up ahead, I would see Ayah sitting outside on the porch, waiting for me. I wanted so badly to be in her arms. I wanted to curl up in her shawl, to cry my tears of rejection and loneliness, to be understood and loved and held in my heartbreak.

There on the hill, Ayah watched me. She didn't move toward me, but she watched. She called me with her eyes. Now that I've been a mother, grandmother, great-grandmother, and great-great-grandmother, I suspect I know what she felt: both heartbreak for me and a deep understanding that things would eventually be all right. She knew I would get through it, even when I didn't. And every day when I arrived at the top of that hill, she would scoop me up, hold me in her shawl, and rock me.

Though I was deep in turmoil, I still had enough energy to want her love. That desire pulled me up the hill and into her arms. It got me through.

If you have nothing else right now, your wanting can get you through, too.

Once you've gotten in touch with your desire, take a moment to connect with the juice you *do* have—even if it feels as if you don't have enough. You might want to close your eyes again, or keep them open and just breathe. Be honest with yourself: What's keeping you going right now? Find one small thing that brings you joy, and let yourself be grateful for it. This will give you the courage you need to go on.

Then ask yourself the bravest questions of all:

What is your current relationship with your juice?

Do you need more of it?

Where could you go, or what could you do, to get it?

Maybe there's something deep inside you that's calling you to try something new. Maybe you want to find paid work that brings you more juice or to get more juice from the work you're already doing. Maybe your juice comes from home. Maybe what gave you juice before is no longer serving, or you need something more. I promise you that whoever you are and wherever you are, there is juice waiting for you if you're able to look for it.

Whether you've lost touch with your juice or have never really given it much thought, you can start by doing something—anything—that feels good. Start small. Think of the thing you identified before, the thing that's keeping you going, and lean into it. Or consider a satisfying project you can tackle in a short amount of time. Make something with your hands, get up and clean behind your sofa, or repot a plant. Remember what it feels like to put your love into action simply for the sake of it.

You can also do something for someone else, such as paint a rock, bake cookies, or practice singing a loved one's favorite song. You don't even need to have someone in mind; trust that if you start making and doing, someone who needs it will come along. If nothing else, everyone can send good energy to others, to think of their happiness and wish them well. These small things may feel insignificant, but they have a remarkable effect.

Juice is at the heart of my first secret because it's where we all start. It's where we end, too, with a life that brings us more and more juice; the rest of my secrets will show you how. But for now, as you're getting started, juice is all you need.

What's most important is to realize that searching for your juice is nearly as important as finding it. The search itself is life reaching for life. Even if you don't have much juice, your longing for more means that some part of you remembers what's possible. It suggests that you are more than just a beating heart—you are a living soul.

Practice: Finding Your Juice

1. First, take a moment to gently put your hand on your heart. Just rest it there, allowing your chest to feel the warmth of your hand, allowing your hand to feel the subtle movement of your heart beating. This is the deepest part of your being. This is where your soul lives. Whenever you fall out of alignment with life, move your hand back to your heart. This simple motion has immense power.

2. Then ask your heart, "What do you love?" Don't just answer it once—repeat the question three or four or ten times. See how your answer evolves as you ask the question over and over.

3. With your hand still on your heart, think back to a time when you felt a sense of purpose. It could be when you achieved something in your profession, when you felt connected to your child, or when you took on a volunteer role. It could also be something small, such as tending to a plant, making a child giggle, or completing an afternoon project. Don't worry if it's been a while since you felt this way; the experience doesn't need to be recent. The point is to remind yourself how you fit into the whole.

4. Then think back to your childhood. Consider your earliest memories of joy and satisfaction. What were you doing? Who were you being? What made your heart sing? What made you giddy with joy? You may get just a fragment or an image. Your unconscious mind knows the answers, but it may speak to you in a symbol or sign, a daydream or dream. You don't need to demand the answer or try to analyze it with your conscious control. Invite your unconscious to tell you when it's ready. It knows.

5. As you explore these memories, feel the sense of meaning attached to them. What did you really love about that action? Why did it feel so good? For instance, maybe you liked helping someone else, or

maybe you enjoyed expressing yourself. Maybe you were surprised by your own talent, or maybe you were able to improve things in a way you found meaningful.

6. Now consider your life today. Is there any small thing you could do that might bring you the same feeling? Imagine yourself moving toward it, exploring it. You can take gradual steps toward finding your juice.

7. When you're finished with the contemplation, find a scrap of paper and write down a word or draw an image that represents some aspect of your juice. Put it somewhere where you will see it often, such as on your bathroom mirror or your fridge, or somewhere where you can carry it with you, such as in your wallet or purse. This is your talisman, your compass. It will help lead you to your juice. Once you know what your heart desires, you will be drawn to fulfill it.

SECRET II

All Life Needs to Move

Chapter 6

FEELING STUCK

Have you ever felt frozen, as if you can't seem to move forward in life? Perhaps it's as if you can't seem to move on from a trauma or a heartbreak—or you can't tap into the passion or enthusiasm that once came so easily. Maybe you're so unmotivated at work that you spend time fantasizing about "getting away" somewhere you can't quite name.

Whatever the cause, you have no idea what to do next—what change to make, what specialist to see.

Or maybe even how to get out of bed.

It's natural for all of us in life, at some point, to feel stuck. Our juice is meant to flow—so what do we do when no matter how hard we try to get more juice, it just seems to stagnate within us?

What can we do about it? How can we respond when it seems as though the world is passing us by and we are just standing still, watching it? Turning toward life requires us to accept what life offers us—but what happens when we feel so exhausted or hurt that we freeze up, unable to open ourselves to what's next?

To answer those questions, let's start by exploring what "stuck" can look like on the physical level.

I once treated a very smart and self-aware eighty-year-old woman who had been suffering from severe intestinal obstructions for several months. Theresa had consulted other doctors and tried everything she knew to do physically, but the blockages had persisted. She came into my office distraught and clearly uncomfortable. "I don't want to live the rest of my life this way," she said.

We started by discussing her diet, which wasn't amazing but wasn't terrible, either. She had altered it significantly to address her constipation, but it hadn't made much of a difference. We then talked about her water intake and how often she exercised. Since nothing seemed off, I then moved on to more holistic questions about her life in a general sense: her emotions, her social support, what brought her days joy and meaning. As she spoke, I noticed that she seemed increasingly closed off to my questions. She paused and looked at me after each question I asked, tightening her lips slightly as if trying to understand my angle before reluctantly offering an answer.

"And what about your dreams?" I asked. "Is your sleeping self trying to tell you anything?"

"My dreams? What would my dreams have to do with it?" Theresa asked, leaning back in her chair and crossing her arms, gripping her upper arms lightly in frustration. She gave me a look that made it clear that she didn't appreciate my deviating from the topic at hand.

The trouble was that from my perspective, those questions had *everything* to do with the topic at hand. Diet, exercise, and hydration are great places to start when it comes to issues affecting digestion. Water is important because it helps break down the food we eat, enabling the body to absorb nutrients. Then water helps what's left to move out. Our diet is crucial because the more whole foods we eat, the more fiber we take in, which helps stimulate our bowels to move food and nutrients through and out of the body. Exercise is important because it increases blood flow to the muscles in and around our gut, helping them do their job. Do you see a pattern here? Our bodies work because they were built to move.

Yet from a holistic perspective, Theresa's problem was pointing to something much bigger. Our digestion is symbolic of how we take in the world and how we let it move through us. Our thoughts and emotions can affect our digestion, too, as they create and release tension around the organs that affect their functioning. So though Theresa didn't particularly want to talk about the rest of her life, I kept trying to get some details about what was going on for her.

Finally, she admitted that she had been feeling sad lately. When I asked why, she reluctantly explained that she had lost someone close to her . . . and someone else . . . and someone else. Eventually, Theresa admitted that she had lost five close friends and family members in the past year. Her eyes flitted toward the ceiling as she said it, then back toward the floor. She looked anywhere but directly into my eyes.

"Have you grieved?" I asked.

She looked at me strangely. "Of course I've grieved. I'm sad."

Something about her answer seemed too simplistic. She seemed to see grief as a reaction, not an experience—as something that *happens*, not something we *do*. Something about her response felt stuck, like her bowel. As we discussed her grief, she became increasingly nervous. I watched her body respond to her emotional state. The effect was undeniable: a tightness came over her, moving through her face, her posture, her fingers, her voice. Her arms were uncrossed by then, but her hands gripped each other in her lap.

That was when I knew that I'd found an opening. To understand how Theresa was digesting food, we first had to look at how she was digesting her experience of loss.

In Western medicine, we don't tend to connect our physical issues to our mental or emotional states. We're trained to look at isolated organs or focus on mechanical issues such as diet and posture, instead of asking patients "What do you think you're holding in your gut?" or "What else in your life isn't working?"

Yet people often know where they're stuck in life, and they can point right to it when questioned.

Theresa's bowel was stuck. But there are many ways for our body to slow down or perhaps even stop completely. Consider an athlete going through a period of her life when she's unable to move because of an injury. Sometimes women's menstrual cycles become irregular or even stop completely during the years when they would otherwise be capable of reproduction.

We can also easily find ourselves stuck psychologically, often due to trauma. Our brain feels as though it's in a loop sometimes *because it actually is*—we've found a well-trodden neural pathway and dug in deep.

We seem to have a deep unconscious knowing that life is supposed to move. This is what makes it so obvious when things are *not* moving—even if we don't yet know what to do about it. This is why it's my second secret: *All life needs to move.* **Life itself is always in movement, so aligning with our life force means that we must always look for the flow within us.**

Though our bodies perform autonomic movement processes, it's important for us to move consciously, as well. A longitudinal study on physical activity and longevity found that even ten minutes of brisk walking daily is associated with a longer life expectancy.[5] Any doctor will tell you that exercise is essential for moving through stress and depression because it signals the brain to release feel-good hormones and that it has profound benefits for physical health in both the long and short term. This is backed by research from around the world indicating that some of the longest life spans are found in cultures where people's lifestyle forces them to walk every day.[6] Exercise helps not only the body but also the mind. It has remarkable positive effects on mood,[7] as well as cognition.[8] It's essential that we integrate movement into our lives.

There are many factors at play here, but to a large extent, much of what the science suggests is simply logical. Stillness promotes tension. And when we hold tension in our body, we restrict our circulation, digestion, and nervous system, making it harder for our body to get nourishment.

In addition, when we don't release emotions and stuck energy, we compromise our lymphatic system, the organs and tissues that fight infection and rid the body of toxins. This is why bodywork is so important and why I myself prioritize receiving massage nearly every week in my stage of life. Though the blood is moved through the body by the heart, lymph has no such organ to move it—it moves when we move, and it stands still when we don't.

A lack of movement also affects our endocrine system, the network of glands that produces and moves hormones to specific tissues and organs in the body. When we get blocked in the adrenal glands, for example, we stay stuck in fear, anger, judgment, and disappointment. We struggle to access the smiles, laughter, and love that can remove the block.

I understand anger to largely be an issue of the adrenals. Righteous anger is a quick and limited reaction to a stimulus, and it proves that the adrenals are working. But chronically overactive adrenals are often related to a type of anger that feels stuck and doesn't move, like a grudge. This can cause a variety of health problems that break the body down faster. Forgiveness allows life to move again, while grudges keep it stuck. Seen through this metaphor, movement is about so much more than pumping our blood and moving our lymph. It's an ethic, a principle, that we can integrate into every aspect of our lives.

And like most of my secrets to health and happiness, it's backed by ancient knowledge. The truth is that no matter how stuck we may find ourselves, *life itself* is always moving. The concept of *anicca*, as it's often transliterated in Buddhist texts, or *anitya*, which is the more common spelling in Hindu texts, is age old. This concept focuses on impermanence: that life is always changing and that suffering comes when we try to stop its flow.

Sometimes this means letting life move through us and around us without trying to stop it. Other times, it means actually getting up and moving ourselves. This applies at the physical, emotional, and spiritual levels. Understanding the power of movement can get us through almost anything. It's a sacred truth that helps us in our hardest moments.

And it starts with realizing that being stuck is itself an illusion.

Chapter 7

LIFE IS ALWAYS MOVING

Let's consider this second secret a little more deeply. All life needs to move—and that means that everything that is alive *is* moving.

That's right: it's moving, even when it's hard to perceive. I liken this to the Arizona desert. I love this landscape. In the more than sixty years I've spent living here, longer than most of you reading this may have been alive, I've seen thousands upon thousands of Sonoran sunsets, the pinks and oranges swirling behind saguaro silhouettes. I've watched families of quail as they hurry into the underbrush, I've watched the prickly pear and ocotillo burst into full flower. Yet many people who come here for the first time—and quite a few more who will never come here in their whole lives—think of this as a still, stagnant, dead place. Boy, are they wrong.

If you think this desert is dead, you've never seen it after the rain.

When monsoon season comes, dark clouds begin to cross the sky every afternoon like clockwork. As they pass overhead, the skies open up, dumping life from above. The rain lasts twenty or thirty minutes at most, and it's over as quickly as it began. That's when the whole ecosystem springs into motion. It was there, alive all the time, just waiting patiently for its moment. The cacti swell up, the birds call out to each other, the lizards run around in jubilation, and all the mice and other little mammals scurry about, looking for puddles to lap up. All of that life is always there; we just don't always perceive it.

Our life force is like that. It's always there, always alive, always moving. It's just waiting for us to notice.

How can I be sure of this? Because I know for certain that when our energy stops moving, we die. That means no matter how stuck we feel, as long as we're alive, something within us is moving. Even when we're sitting still, each of us is our own universe of motion. Something is always shifting, even if it isn't flowing particularly well. As long as we're alive, our hearts beat. Our lungs take in air and push it out again. Our digestive system works continuously—even if it's painfully slow. It is in our very nature to move, to process, to release. Motion is happening through us, within us, and around us.

This simple principle works on many levels. As emotional and spiritual beings, we can't thrive when we focus on what's stuck— whether it be a thought, feeling, identity, diagnosis, point of view, or even person. That's because our stuckness holds no life.

When we connect with the idea of movement, we tap into something our body does naturally. Not only are our organs, tissues, and fluids designed to move, but our energy is, too. This is true not only on a visible level—in sweat, digestion, and other physical processes— but also on an invisible level.

Children understand this. That's why they're always wiggling. I never stopped wiggling, in part because I couldn't, and in part because I never saw anything wrong with it. I never taught my children to stop wiggling, either. Wiggling is good for us—it indicates that life is happening around and through us. It moves our lymph, lubricates our joints, and keeps our muscles from getting tight.

When we feel joy in our body, wiggling, walking, and moving around are natural responses. The inverse is also true: wiggling, walking, and moving around can help us feel more joyful. A brisk walk is incredibly helpful for the brain, which doesn't like us to sit still, either.

This concept of energy flow has been studied for millennia in the East, on an even subtler scale. Traditional Chinese medicine is based on an understanding of energy flow that runs to and from specific organs through *meridians,* or energy channels that run through the body. Treatments such as acupuncture, acupressure, and moxibustion are applied to key points on these meridians to unblock them, activate them, and help the energy flow. In the 1970s, Bill and I became early adopters of acupuncture in the allopathic community. Though acupuncture is an ancient science that has been practiced for thousands of years, until recently it was relatively unknown in Western medicine, and doctors ridiculed the Chinese practice of sticking needles into people, comparing it to bloodletting and other antiquated and outdated allopathic practices. They weren't the least bit curious about *why* traditional Chinese medical doctors were doing what they were doing, in some cases because they couldn't imagine it, in others because they were closed-minded and had succumbed to prejudice. I first came to understand a little bit more about acupuncture from a response to a letter Bill and I printed in our newsletter, *Pathways to Health.* A man wrote in that he had applied a treatment to his neck, addressing a specific symptom, and received remarkable benefits in his ankle, where he was experiencing another symptom entirely. He wanted to know how it had happened.

Remember, that was before Google. There weren't online forums to consult or any other places to post a question like that. Our little newsletter, which we printed each month in our clinic and mailed to subscribers around the globe, was many people's best source of information about natural and integrative health. Bill and I were learning right along with everyone else, and we had no idea why treating the man's neck would affect his ankle. We printed the letter verbatim and asked if anyone could explain it. Right away, a doctor wrote in all the way from Italy to say that both points were on the same meridian.

At the time, I had never heard of meridians, so I started gathering information the old-school way: by reading and asking around. The more I learned, the more sense it made. But I needed more information than I could get locally or through letters, so I decided to bring the information to me. In 1973, Bill and I hosted the United States' first symposium on acupuncture. We held it at Stanford University in California and invited thought leaders in the field of acupuncture from all over the world. President Richard Nixon had just gone to China and had witnessed an appendectomy in which pain relief had been managed with acupuncture alone, without anesthesia. President Nixon's physician, Dr. Paul Dudley White, attended our symposium, as did 280 other medical doctors. Bill and I were among the first MDs to promote the study of acupuncture in the Western medical community, as we started hosting conferences and bringing speakers in from China and around the world. Soon after that, I began treating people with it myself and was astonished by the quick results.

Early in my journey with acupuncture, I was attending the labor of a teenage girl who was terrified to give birth. She was all alone, with no partner to support her, and quite young. She cried through each of her contractions, knowing that the pain would only grow more intense and fearing what was to come. I felt truly bad for her. I also worried that a child was being born into an atmosphere of deep emotional suffering. I have always been a proponent of loving birth, and though I didn't blame the mother for her fear or her pain, I knew that both she and her child deserved a more positive experience.

I asked my patient whether she would be open to allowing me to treat her with acupuncture. She agreed, though she was skeptical. I put needles into a set of points that I had learned were beneficial for labor and sat at her side. Slowly, her tears began to dry, and her breathing became heavier as she relaxed. After a few minutes, I was surprised to find that she'd fallen asleep! She passed many hours like that, waking up for each contraction and falling back asleep between them. By tapping into her meridians, she was able to tap into the flow of life. That comforted and relaxed her. Her energy started to move, and she could focus on something beyond her pain and fear.

Life is always moving; we just need to notice it. It's moving through our meridians. It's moving through our heartbeat. Understanding this is simply a matter of expanding our focus.

Consider life flowing like a forest stream. A tree falls across the stream, creating a small dam, and some sticks come along to build the dam up a little higher. Downstream of the dam, the water flow may slow significantly, but it usually doesn't stop completely. Even if it does, the water continues to flow upstream of the dam, and the movement can be seen in the rising waterline. At some point, the water reaches the top of the dam and a trickle forms on one side or another, going around the dam and continuing downstream. If we look only at the dam and the water pooled behind it, we may think that the water has stopped—but it's always moving.

Life reaches for life. Always. That means that when we feel the most stuck, whether physically, emotionally, situationally, or any other way, we need only to look for where things are still moving. When we put our focus and our energy there, a trickle will form around our dam. Aligning with this trickle will help us realign with life.

When we do, we can get up and start moving again. Once that happens, all we need to do is keep going.

Nowadays, many of us have digital trackers that tell us how many steps we take, and we can set goals to reach. I am no exception; during the long months of Covid quarantine, I challenged myself to continue getting my 3,700 steps a day, and many times I do it simply by walking around and around my kitchen table. I've kept up my pace since the world opened up again, and lately, I've even increased my daily goal to 3,800 steps! Lucky for me, my home is filled with treasures from my travels around the world. I look at them as I move, remembering the places I've been and the people I've met. The shelves that line my walls hold stones picked up from mountain paths and seashells from the beaches of distant shores. On the wall, I see pictures of my various family members: my parents in the 1930s, myself in the 1940s, my youngest two children posing for a Christmas card in the 1960s, my daughter Analea posing for her high school yearbook in the 1970s, forty years prior to her death. I see crystals and wind chimes, trinkets given to me by patients and friends over the course of many decades, and awards that have honored me in a long and meaningful career. I may be at home, but I don't feel stuck.

This seems so simple, but it can be challenging, especially when our bodies get used to *not* moving and we become physically weak, physically injured, or emotionally depressed.

Chapter 8

MOVING THROUGH PAIN

In the years of the baby boom, we didn't have a term to describe the common experience of young mothers whose body, brain chemistry, and sense of identity were railroaded by early motherhood—a condition that today we'd call *postpartum depression*. But named or not, in the small town on the banks of the Ohio River where Bill and I started our family, the situation was all too common.

There weren't a lot of opportunities in that town. Most people were low income, and few had access to higher education. Beyond that, it was a different time, and women's opportunities were limited beyond the socioeconomic conditions of the region. Many of those young women had done everything expected of them. It was common for them to have married their high school sweethearts and gotten pregnant right away, often having several children in quick succession. That was before the legalization of "the pill," which was what we all called birth control at the time, and in any case it was expected that married women wanted to be pregnant and stay home. I don't know whether Maria did or not; I don't think she knew, either.

She came to see me for headaches that were keeping her on the couch most of the day. She had brought two babies with her—

one she jiggled on her hip in my office, his dark curls bouncing to the rhythm as his bright eyes gazed out the window, and the other crawled around on the floor, dirtying her knees as she explored the corners in a way that made the messy little girl in me proud. As I did with many of my patients, I began by asking Maria about her life.

She told me she loved fashion magazines and spent most of her days reading them and dreaming of another life. Though Maria's sister, cousins, and school friends were all in similar situations and didn't live far away, she rarely reached out to them, and over time they had just stopped calling. "I feel like I just *can't* get up," she explained. "It's like something is pressing me down, and then this terrible headache comes on at about two or three o'clock every day. But by then I have to get up anyway, because I have to clean up and get to cooking before my husband comes home." Just then her daughter, who was lying on her back under the table, sat up suddenly, hitting her head. She burst into tears. Within seconds, her younger brother was crying, too.

I reached down for the little girl as Maria began to bounce and soothe her son, but for several minutes, the room was full of their wailing. With four little ones at home, I knew the situation well and wasn't bothered. But looking over at Maria, I could see she'd just about had it. Her eyes widened, and her jaw twisted into a false smile. "Hush now, everything is all right," she whispered unconvincingly as she bounced, with the type of desperation specific to young parents. Finally the children stopped crying—and that was when Maria's own tears started.

She looked at me with the same beautiful dark eyes as her son, wet with tears. "Oh, Dr. Gladys, do you think I'm a terrible mother?" I didn't think Maria was a terrible mother; I thought she was depressed.

"What are the kids doing while you're on the sofa?" I asked her.

"You know, they're kids. They're pointing at the pictures in a book. They're snuggling their teddy bear. They're pressing the buttons on their toys until something pops out."

"And are you moving at all?"

"No."

"Are you sure?"

I explained the dam and the trickle to Maria. I told her about the desert after the rain. Then I told her that she was moving, too—in some way or another. She just had to notice it.

"I'd like to suggest that you *are* moving, and you just need to grab onto your movement and keep going with it. At the very least, you're breathing and you're turning the pages of your magazine. Take that movement and go with it."

Maria was confused. "What, do you mean, turn the pages *faster*?"

"No—as you're turning the page, let your whole arm move. Let that little movement of turning the page become a bigger movement in which you use your arm and shoulder. Use that momentum. Get up, walk around the house, look outside. It may be that you notice a butterfly through the window and you walk toward it, or you see some wildflowers to go pick in the yard. Just don't let yourself sit there, frozen. At some point, your mind will start to follow your body. You'll see something beautiful or inspiring, and you'll align with the light once again."

Maria's eyes narrowed as she continued to bounce the baby. She was unconvinced.

"See how you're bouncing that baby there?" I asked, and she nodded. "Bounce yourself, Maria. You need it as much as he does. Even when you can't get off the couch, see if you can sit there and shake for a whole minute without stopping. Start there."

On my lap, the little girl had taken off one shoe and sock and was inspecting her toes. I reached down for her big toe, grabbed it, and said, "This little piggy went to the market . . . " she squealed in delight, knowing what was coming next. I gently pinched her second toe between my fingers and began to work my way down toward the pinky. "This little piggy stayed home. This little piggy had roast beef, this little piggy had none. And this little piggy went '*Wheeeeeee!!!*' all the way home!" She rocked her body as I tickled her belly, both of us giggling.

When I looked back to Maria, she was smiling, though her eyes were still quizzical.

"It isn't easy to be a mother," I said softly.

She nodded, the tears welling up again.

"But you need these silly little games as much as they do. You need to laugh with them, to reach for them, to move with them—not because it will make you a good mother, but because it will allow you to survive. You've got to get those giggles in and keep moving. Otherwise, it's just dirty diapers forever." Maria leaned toward me, and I scooted my chair closer. Then I held her, the two children cradled between us, as she released a flood of tears.

I knew her situation was desperate, so I was as surprised as anyone when my solution alone pulled her out of it. Maria got moving, and she started accessing her life force again. When I saw her several months later, she was regularly meeting a cousin for walks to the playground. They would push their little babies on the swings—sometimes even swinging themselves—and commiserate about the challenges of motherhood. Eventually, Maria started sketching her own fashion designs and expressing herself creatively at her kitchen table. She found a way to make motherhood work for her.

Today, I might offer someone like Maria different resources. Perhaps a similar patient would get mental health support from a licensed therapist or use psychiatric medications to get her out of her hole. If her headaches were diagnosed as migraines or cluster headaches, medications for those might also be useful. She might go to a gym to get her endorphins flowing, instead of just shaking and walking around the neighborhood. But even today, when we have more resources available, we often have to get moving to access them—we have to awaken our life force in order to ask for help. And believe it or not, wandering around the house or playing "This little piggy" with a baby is better than sitting frozen on the couch.

Depression is insidious. It's invasive and sneaky, like a virus. It creeps in undetected, until all of a sudden it's there, fully present, and we don't know what to do about it. When that happens, we need to find simple ways to connect with our lives again.

It can be hard to get moving when we're depressed. It can also be hard when we're in great pain. But the emotional pain of depression is very similar to physical pain, and often, as much as it may hurt, movement is part of the solution to pain.

Another patient of mine, Suzy, had rheumatoid arthritis and lived with pain every day. She was excited to become pregnant, but I was concerned that she would suffer even more, particularly during labor. Her joints were inflamed as part of her arthritis. Pregnancy puts pressure on joints, releasing hormones that cause them to expand further than they otherwise would, and birth itself increases both those hormones and that pressure. I knew that labor involves some of the greatest pain most women will ever experience; that would be even more true for someone with rheumatoid arthritis. She wanted to go through the experience without intervention, including medication, yet I worried about how she could accomplish it.

I was lucky enough to attend Suzy as she gave birth. Like any laboring woman, she was in pain, and I knew that hers was greater than most. But in that precious portal between worlds, in the deep universal knowing that women are so often blessed with while in labor, she seemed to know precisely what to do. Something primal took place before my eyes. That amazing woman, who was used to the challenge of living with chronic pain, somehow allowed herself to be moved by what hurt. She stopped fighting, and she let it take her over completely.

As each contraction came, gripping her in its ferocity, she surrendered her entire body to it. I watched as her movements slowly built to a rhythm and then to a dance. She swirled slowly through the room, her bare feet on the floor, swaying her hips like an ancient goddess, like a *woman who knows*. I will never forget watching that incredible woman dance her way through birth, welcoming her daughter into the world by moving with the pain. The pain was of course very real, but at the same time, she didn't cling to it. She let it be transient. In that way, she opened herself to great joy. The transient pain morphed into transcendental bliss as she welcomed her child into the world through a healthy and loving birth.

I stood back in utter awe. Though I have witnessed hundreds, if not thousands, of births in my lifetime, I continue to be amazed by its miracle.

Suzy was tapping into something much greater than herself—a wisdom that reaches back through the generations.

Scientific studies show us that many types of chronic pain are helped by movement.[9] Movement keeps our joints lubricated and healthy. It keeps our muscles from deteriorating so they can support our ligaments and bones. It keeps our blood circulating. And it gives us something to focus on besides the pain itself.

So how should we move when we're in pain? As counterintuitive as it may seem, the answer is quite simple: we should just move any way. Of course, there are exceptions—such as when we have a spinal injury or a bone that is setting—but most of the time, some sort of movement is possible, even if we have to keep the part of our body that hurts still. And movement also fends off the depression that can keep us even more stuck.

Fear is one of the major reasons we stop moving as a response to pain: we don't want to hurt more. But since life is always in movement, movement is always there. If you're in pain, start with deepening your breathing. Notice how that moves your belly and chest. Allow your body to start moving with the breath, making it bigger and bigger. You may notice that the pain ebbs and flows as you do. You may notice that moving this way or that makes it more bearable. And you may even find yourself starting to rise up and move more. Follow that and see what happens. Who knows? You may even start dancing.

If you live with chronic pain, you'll find that moving through it will eventually become a habit. If your mind tends toward depression, you can also learn to get moving when you feel a depressive episode arising.

Sometimes there is a physical reason for our pain: we may have been injured in the past, or we may have inherited brain chemistry that leads toward unstable moods. Other times, it's past experiences that lead to stagnation. That's why it's important to consider the role of shame, the body's most paralyzing emotion.

Chapter 9

LOCKED IN SHAME

Shame is one of the hardest emotions to release. Many people live their whole lives held in its grip. We're often particularly plagued by old shame—situations that repeat themselves over and over again, as much as we wish they didn't. Nothing contracts our life force more than shame.

Everyone experiences shame at one time or another. For reasons that aren't fully clear to me, I have a strong pattern of slipping and falling onstage. It's embarrassing, but it just happens! Though thinking back to those incidents still causes a little twinge, I've learned to transform it into humor. That seems to defang the embarrassing incidents.

The first time I had a public fall, I was in elementary school. I was proud to be playing the lead role in the school play called *The Frog Jumped over the Pool*. I stood in my green costume, prepared for the seminal moment: my triumphant leap over a dishpan full of water. The crowd watched. But something went wrong midway through the air, and I ended up first hearing, and then feeling, the water splash beneath me. There I sat in the dishpan as the crowd roared with laughter, green dye bleeding from my frog suit and into the water, paralyzed with humiliation and crying hysterically.

Later, as my brothers told the story at our dinner table, my mother recognized a teachable moment. She waited for my brothers to stop laughing before saying "All right, boys, now that you've had your fun, what can we do as a family to help Gladee so that the next time she feels embarrassed, she can help people laugh *with* her instead of *at* her?" She said it with utter love and compassion—for my embarrassment and also for the absurdity of the situation. She didn't shame me for crying, but she didn't shame my brothers for laughing, either.

It turned out that her question held its own answer. When we release the shame of being the one in the pool, we realize what everyone else already knows: it actually *is* quite funny to attend a play called *The Frog Jumped over the Pool*, only to have that promise go splashing into a dishpan. If we let embarrassment move, it often turns into something else—in this case, humor.

That lesson served me several times over because it turned out to only be the first of many occasions when I fell onstage. In college, I took a class called Public Speaking 101. Every student had to go up and introduce herself in front of the others. I was nervous because I was already quite different from the other girls, having recently moved to Ohio from India. As I walked up to the podium to introduce myself, I tripped on the step and fell flat on my behind. Before the *boom* of my landing, two other loud sounds ricocheted through the room: the *crack* of my head on the desk, and the *rip* of my skirt splitting to above the knee, which at the time was quite risqué. Remembering my mother's lesson from the school play, I quickly recovered myself and released my embarrassment. Then, while the audience was still gasping with shock, I announced, "The first thing a speaker must do is get the attention of the audience. My name is Gladys Taylor, and I hope you enjoyed the show!" The audience roared with laughter—as did I.

Understanding that life needs to move works just like that: we recognize what isn't working, and we let it go to see what else is there. In that case, when I released my humiliation for having made a mistake, I found the humor lying beyond it. That humor brought me nothing but joy, and it simply would not have been available to me if I had remained stuck in my shame and embarrassment. I had to first forgive myself for making a mistake. Then the energy could start to move again.

That was what my mother was trying to teach me. When I sat in the pan of water crying, I wasn't crying because I'd fallen—I was an active kid, and I fell all the time. I was crying because I thought that I *shouldn't have* fallen and I was ashamed. Consider Maria and Suzy, whom you met in the previous chapter. My frozen shame onstage is similar to Maria's fear that she wasn't a good mother. And it highlights what Suzy *didn't* do during her labor—she didn't sit there worrying about her arthritis and her difficult labor, thinking something wasn't right about the situation. That would have distracted her from the job she had to do, which was birth the baby. She just got moving and let life and love—and even laughter—flow through her.

My mother taught me to laugh when I feel shame because laughter has an uncanny ability to break right through what hurts. In the body, laughter serves an important purpose. It quite literally tickles the adrenals. The diaphragm is located just above the adrenal glands, which house our reactivity, our fear and anger, our apathy and hatred. When we laugh, we flex and release the diaphragm. This gives a light jiggle to the adrenals that I think of as a tickle. "Hey, there," it says, "are you feeling stressed or upset? Is there anything you'd like to release?" In my experience, the adrenals are often quite relieved by the invitation to relax and let go.

Shame is one of the most stagnant emotions we carry as humans. At the dinner table, my mother showed me that instead of locking up with embarrassment, I could find an emotion that was *in motion* and ride it right on out of my shame.

Now, if you think emotions such as shame and embarrassment disappear with old age, I can promise you that you're wrong! I still have the opportunity to release embarrassing moments, even at 103.

I had one such opportunity on my ninety-ninth birthday. I was still driving at the time, and I stopped by the supermarket to pick up a few things. Out at my car, I was lifting my bag of groceries in the way that a ninety-nine-year-old woman would: slowly. I guess it attracted some attention, because an elderly gentleman came over to assist me.

"Would you like some help?" he asked.

"Oh, thank you, but I'm just fine," I said.

"Really, I can help you. I'm stronger than I look. I'm eighty-six!" he said proudly.

Something about that irked me. I don't know why, but it did. And somehow I heard myself spitting out a nasty retort: "Hmmph. Well, I'm ninety-nine!" I stared directly at him as I said it, challenging him with my eyes.

He was a bit taken aback by my response. Then he said something else in a friendly tone and walked away. I closed the back of the car and sat down in the driver's seat, fuming at myself. Why had I said something so unpleasant? Why had I felt competitive with him? He'd only wanted to help! "You're becoming a nasty old woman, Gladys," I thought to myself. I felt too upset to start the car.

Then I thought, "What about this situation could be seen as funny?" And suddenly, I saw it: two old people snapping at each other in a supermarket parking lot. That was funny! An old woman treating a man of eighty-six like a young whippersnapper. That was funny, too! The more I looked at the situation, the more it appeared like a scene from a comedy show, with two grumpy senior citizens griping at each other over a bag of groceries. I sat in that car and tickled my adrenals until my belly hurt. Somehow it became too ridiculous to be embarrassing anymore. I released my shame and my regret, had a laugh, and let it go.

The next time you find yourself doing something embarrassing, I encourage you to try to think about how it could be seen as funny. What about your mistake is humorous? What was surprising, silly, or just plain ridiculous? How would someone on the outside see it, and why might they laugh? You'll be surprised by how often a humorous interpretation is available if you only go looking for it.

This trick works easily with small incidents like the one I just described. But often, the thing that we hold on to is regret about the bigger choices we make in life. How can we release our feelings about bigger decisions we've made in the past: the relationships we've lost, the financial decisions we navigated poorly, the career choices gone awry?

Finding movement also includes forgiving ourselves for what we did not know or did not do better in the past.

Chapter 10

RELEASING WHAT DOESN'T MATTER

Throughout our lives, many of us struggle with feeling stuck on an idea or experience. When truly challenging events arrive, they deserve processing, and it often feels as though our entire being dedicates itself to getting through something. Yet sometimes we seem to get stuck in this processing. Sometimes we can't manage to move on.

There's a fine line between moving on and flat-out denial, but I believe we all know what the difference feels like. Most of us know when a process has been obstructed. This is when we ruminate, considering the same thought over and over again or almost torturing ourselves with a memory we can't seem to release. It's when something we loved, such as a relationship, career path, or project, comes to an end and we find ourselves lamenting what we no longer have instead of building things anew. When this happens, we sometimes need a quick release. We need to look at what is no longer serving us and simply let it go.

Most of us also know what it feels like to come up against something that isn't going to serve us at all. Being open to life sometimes means turning away from things that aren't good for us. We can say a kind but firm "No, thank you" and just keep going on with our lives.

My mother had a profound understanding of this principle. My sister Margaret and I were already old ladies when we looked at each other one day and noticed that we both make a funny hand gesture when we speak. We raise our hand gently in front of us, fingers held loosely, palm up. Then we swoop it down and back, as though we're releasing flower petals into flowing water beneath us. *What in the world is going on with that?* we wondered. *Who started that trend?*

Then we both remembered: "Mama did it."

She'd make that gesture and say, "*Kutch par wa nay,*" Hindustani for "It doesn't matter." That was how our mother taught us to let things go. For her, it was a natural movement. It was what enabled her to live through immense challenges without letting them in too deeply; she just released what wasn't working, refocused on what was important to her, and moved on. My mother was never gruff or callous; she was deeply compassionate. Yet she also had important work to do in this world, and *kutch par wa nay* enabled her to continue to do it.

Throughout my life, I've found this to be a useful practice. I've done it for years—long before Margaret and I even realized what it was. I would recognize something that didn't serve me and drop my hand, opening my fingers in a fluid motion to signify its release. Now that the gesture has become conscious, I realize that there's great empowerment in knowing that whenever I notice something coming toward me, I can choose whether to take it in. And if it's something I don't want, I consciously give the energy back to wherever it came from. I don't hold it tight and static in my hand. I recognize that the universe is moving, and I release it back like flowers in the water.

It seems that I'm never short of opportunities to practice *kutch par wa nay*. I also like to use it when I come up against emotions that I need to feel and transform. It's particularly effective when dealing with regret.

I've regretted plenty of decisions in my life, which means I've had plenty of opportunities to learn how to forgive myself. I've regretted things I've said, people I've hurt, and choices I've made. I've also regretted opinions I've held. But I refuse to hold on to my regret.

Over the course of a century, my knowledge has grown significantly—just as I hope yours has and will continue to do during your lifetime. My opinions have evolved, too. This is a natural part of being alive.

There are things I used to think were right that I now think are wrong. It's true; no matter how strong you are in your convictions today, if you live more than a hundred years, I'm sure there are ideas and opinions you hold now that you, too, will come to disagree with! One of the things I've really struggled with relates to my career. It affected hundreds of women and children who were in my care during some of the most vulnerable moments of their lives.

Back when I was trained to deliver babies, the common understanding was that women should be put into what was called a "twilight sleep" to avoid the pain of labor. Then, because the woman was unable to push, the doctor would extract the baby with forceps.

I gave birth to my first two children that way. I delivered many others with forceps, myself, and I was even pretty good at it. I did it because I was taught that that way of doing things was an absolute godsend after centuries of women going through the excruciating pain of giving birth. At the time, it seemed like a compassionate, woman-centered view. I now see it as a brutal way to welcome a baby into the world—one that is largely unnecessary.

Today, although I support women who want pain medication during birth, I think it's just plain wrong to tell women that they can't do it on their own. I recognize the power and importance of going through the birthing process, and whether women end up having a high-intervention birth or not, I would never suggest that they should be drugged reflexively. I also think it's traumatic to a baby to be pulled out by the head.

Looking back, I suppose I could blame myself for the births I attended this way. I could blame myself for the way I gave birth to my first two children, too. It wasn't the way I chose to give birth to the children who were born later.

This extends to far more than birthing; I could blame myself for the foods I fed my children when I thought they were healthy, the opinions I formed that I now find shocking, or the things I said that I would love to take back. But I could also just say "*Kutch par wa nay*" and know that after I received different information, I behaved differently. I mostly did the best I could with what I had at the time. I made the choices I made with love, and I choose to live without regret. Everyone faces regret—the question is, how long should we hold on to it?

Back in that Ohio town, I once worked with a father who quite nearly killed his own newborn baby by accident. Matthew was maybe twenty years old, and his wife, Connie, was even younger. I'd treated Connie throughout her pregnancy and knew she was near to term. But like a lot of people in the area, she labored for a good long while before they called me, and it took me a bit of time to get there.

It was a busy time. When we started our practice, we were two of six general practitioners in town, but one by one the rest had all retired. Then Bill went into the service during the Korean War. That left me alone caring for nearly nine thousand patients, along with the four young children I was raising. I was treating another patient when I got the call, and it took me about an hour to wrap things up and make it out into the hills to Connie's home.

Matthew answered the door in panic. "Dr. Gladys, Connie done had the baby already, and she's bleeding an awful lot."

"Who's bleeding?" I asked, rushing to pull off my gloves and hat as I hurried down the hall with my doctor's bag. "Connie or the baby?"

"Well, both," he said, his face pale, "but it's the baby I'm worried about. I cut that cord like I was supposed to and blood's just gushing out."

I pushed through the door to the bedroom, where I saw Connie white with fright, holding a small bundle in her arms. There was a good deal of mess from the birth on the sheets, and a pair of scissors was left open on the nightstand. I reached down for the baby and saw that the blanket was stained red. No one said a word as I peeled it back. There, the tiny belly was covered in blood—gushing was the right word for it, as her cord had been cut flush with the skin. The newborn was as silent as her parents, which chilled me to the bone.

Normally, we clamp the cord before we cut it an inch or two in front of the belly button. This helps the umbilical artery, which until this point has been responsible for the baby's blood supply, to close. There's an ugly stump for a few days that eventually falls off. And in any case, there's no need to cut the cord right away. But Matthew, coursing with adrenaline after delivering his daughter and uneducated about what to do next, had thought of his own belly button cut right to the base and had cut his daughter's just the same.

I reached into my medical bag for my tools, found a small set of forceps called hemostats, and doused them in disinfectant. The baby had lost a lot of blood, and there was no time to waste. Matthew and Connie held each other, gasping, as I kneeled down next to the bed and dug around in the newborn's belly, looking for the umbilical artery. It was deep in there, and the infant started to scream just as soon as I touched the wound, raising to a desperate screech as I prodded around with my hemostats. When she stopped screaming, I worried even more. She was so weak from the loss of blood that she could no longer cry. It took what felt like several agonizing minutes for me to get hold of that artery, while that baby first hollered and then panted, but I grabbed it, clamped it, and saved her life.

Later, Matthew tried to apologize, but I shushed him as quickly as he started. "Matthew, you did the absolute best you could with the information you had," I said kindly but firmly. "Don't you go wasting your energy on this—your wife and child need you now. Of course it was an accident. Of course you didn't know. There's no sense beating yourself up for something that can't be helped." I dropped my hand toward the floor as I said, "Let it go. Your daughter is alive, and she's going to be fine. Just let it go." And I was right. I knew their family for several years after that, and the little girl was just fine.

I've thought about him for years, that young, scared father up in the hills delivering a baby on his own. I've prayed that the mistake didn't haunt him, because I believe what I said: there's no sense beating ourselves up for something that can't be helped. The best thing we can do is release it and move on.

I don't know what mistakes you've made in the past, but I'd like to suggest that you, too, mostly did the best you could with what you had at the time. If you find yourself living with regret, try to catch it and see what's moving. Did things mostly turn out all right? If so, be grateful! Is there anything funny about it? If so, laugh! Have you learned anything new since then? If so, enjoy what you now know and express it however you can! Do whatever you can do to let your regret go—forgive yourself and, if necessary, ask for forgiveness from others—so you can move on with your life.

Sometimes we find that a simple action such as saying "*Kutch par wa nay*" can make all the difference. But on occasion, we hold on to regret, pain, or perceived stuckness because there's a block in our system that we need to remove.

Chapter 11

REMOVING THE BLOCKAGE

There are times in life and health when healing can occur only when an actual blockage is removed. We often have a deep knowing when this is the case—when a certain food we're eating, relationship we're engaging in, or pattern in our life needs to be removed.

In many cases, it's simply a belief. That was true for my patient, Shanti. Shanti was pregnant and intent on having an intervention-free birth. She was a seasoned spiritual practitioner, so she had meditated and done a good deal of spiritual work to prepare herself for labor. The trouble was that she hadn't done any of the physical exercises that I and the nurse midwife, Barbara Brown, had prescribed her. When it came time for her to go into labor, she languished at one centimeter dilation. Her cervix wasn't open nearly enough for her to begin to push, and after many hours of contractions, I worried that she was becoming too tired to continue.

Shanti was closed to a lot of the ideas we had given her, just as she was closed to interventions in her birth. To put it kindly, she was a person who liked to do things her way, every time. It struck me that her mind was as unable to open as her cervix was. In my desire to help I became frustrated, so I decided to get moving. I left the room for a few minutes to collect my thoughts while Barbara assisted her. As I paced around the house, not wanting to be out of earshot in case there was a problem, I found myself wondering *Where is life moving? Where can I work with the flow that is already happening?*

Barbara figured out what I couldn't. She remembered that Shanti liked to chant as part of her spiritual practice, so she suggested that they start chanting together. Out in the hallway, I heard their voices coming through the bedroom door: "Open lotus, lotus open. Open lotus, lotus open." Barbara tapped into an area where the patient was open-minded. She recognized the blockage: that there was physical work to be done, as well as spiritual work. So instead of focusing on the blockage, she got the energy flowing around spirituality, and from there, Shanti's cervix physically opened. But despite being fully dilated, Shanti didn't want to push. So Barbara changed the chant to "Down and out," and with a few pushes the baby showed her face. Shortly thereafter, Shanti held a healthy baby in her arms—birthed, as she'd hoped, entirely without medical intervention.

Remember, when we find ourselves stuck, we need to look for the trickle going around the dam. For Shanti, it was through the spiritual work that she already knew and was comfortable doing. That allowed things to shift for her. In that shift, she found movement, and what was blocking her was able to be released.

Sometimes what's blocking us requires us to make a big change. After years of fighting for things to go her way, my friend Elisabeth Kübler-Ross eventually removed her own blockage: she let her fight go and moved clear across the country.

Elisabeth and I had known each other as colleagues for years. Her background bore similarities to my own. She had been born in Switzerland and had gone on to conduct and publish groundbreaking research on grief. Her breakout best seller, *On Death and Dying*, was published in 1969 and is still in print today. It outlines five stages of grief, which Elisabeth explained as nonconsecutive phases we move through as we grieve.

In the 1980s, Elisabeth was moved by the tragic deaths of those who had contracted AIDS. At the time, it was known as the "AIDS crisis," and there was a lot of stigma around the people who contracted it because many of them were gay men. In the early days of AIDS there were many children who contracted it, too, either through blood transfusions, through birth from an HIV-positive mother, or through sexual abuse. Elisabeth wanted to open a hospice center near her newly purchased home in rural Virginia for children who had contracted it. Many of the children's parents had abandoned them, and Elisabeth found that unconscionable.

But some of her neighbors were so homophobic they couldn't even feel badly for these kids. They thought that AIDS was synonymous with homosexuality and worried that openly gay people would move to Virginia and disrupt the conservative community living there. Others just didn't want to contract HIV themselves, and they didn't have a reasonable understanding of how it spread. Elisabeth fought for her hospice center and lost, but the community never fully forgave her for being so avant-garde.

I remember talking to her about it—it made her hopping mad that the community had moved against her hospice plan. She was upset that people were homophobic, a prejudice that had never made sense to either of us, and she felt it was even more ridiculous that their fear and hatred had extended to a bunch of sick kids who had nothing to do with homosexuality. But she wanted to stay in Virginia anyway; she was determined to find her way in the community and even hoped she could be a leader for other progressive thinkers who might want to move there.

Then strange things began to happen, leading Elisabeth to believe that someone was targeting her. Some years after her attempt at opening the hospice center, her fears were confirmed. First her home and office were burglarized, and she found bullet holes in the sign to her teaching center. Then one night when she was out of town, someone sneaked onto her property, killed her beloved pet llama, and set her house on fire. It burned to the ground.

Elisabeth was devastated. Though she'd tried to ignore the hostility toward her in the community, she knew it was time to leave. Trying to be herself—leading workshops on grief and supporting the social justice movements that were important to her—was just too hard where she lived. She was sick of trying to prove that she wasn't that different or that scary, so she sold the property and moved out to Scottsdale.

I suppose that from one angle, that could be read as a tragic response to aggression. But I didn't see it that way, nor did Elisabeth herself. Though she was hurt and angry at the people who had pushed her out, she didn't run from them; instead, she courageously chose to take the moment when she'd lost everything as a sign that there was something better waiting for her. Since she had been traveling when her house had burned down, everything she owned fit into a single suitcase. She treated it as an opportunity: to start anew, to be reborn, to make what she could out of a difficult situation.

Sometimes you move somewhere and realize it's not the right place. Sometimes a dream job turns out to be a nightmare. Sometimes a relationship cannot be salvaged and needs to end. These are major life decisions, and no one can make them for you. You are the only one who knows the difference between running away from and running toward in your own life. You are the only one who can say for sure whether you're avoiding something difficult or simply letting go of something that is no longer serving you.

In the years after Elisabeth moved to Scottsdale, she and I went from being colleagues to being dear friends. The arson in Virginia was never solved. And though it remained a point of pain for Elisabeth, she found rich and beautiful things in her years in Arizona. She became a vibrant part of this community, and she continued to advocate for people living with HIV and AIDS. She removed the block by making a change, letting it go, and moving on with her life.

Focusing on the community she wanted to create was key to that process. Elisabeth had hoped to gather others with progressive ideas about spirituality and medicine in rural Virginia, which resembled her homeland in Switzerland. A similar community was already forming in Arizona. By focusing on the community she wanted, Elisabeth clarified her intention, and when it was time to leave Virginia for good, she knew exactly where to go.

When we're stuck and something is blocking us, it is immensely helpful to clarify what it is that we want. This helps us get our energy moving again. It helps us understand exactly what is and isn't working. Eventually, even in a situation as violent and difficult as Elisabeth's, it's this sort of movement that will set us free.

For Elisabeth, the community she dreamed of was what began to form a trickle around the dam.

Chapter 12

LOOK FOR THE TRICKLE
AROUND THE DAM

In chapter 9, I explained that life is always moving—there's always a trickle forming around the dam.

When we focus on this trickle, we start to notice life's natural movement. As we move through our pain, be it physical, emotional, or spiritual, we begin to relax our shame, maybe even laugh about it, and release it along with everything else that isn't serving us. The trickle begins to grow, eventually bursting the dam that blocks us. The impossible becomes possible, and we find ourselves rising to meet our own life force in ways we never imagined.

This is often the case with grief. Grief isn't quite the same as depression—grief moves, while depression stands still. When we let our grief move, we don't suppress it; instead, we focus on our love for whomever or whatever was lost, while letting the suffering pass through us. The goal isn't to get rid of our grief or to make it go away faster, nor is it to hold on to it forever and ever. Yet the moment grief separates from the principle of movement, it can become stuck. As Elisabeth's important research shows us, we have to keep moving between the stages, allowing our truth and our grief to flow.

How can you help someone who seems stuck in the suffering of grief? Start by creating a safe space and getting the person talking. Every once in a while, this alone can cause the dam to break.

This was the case for Theresa, the patient who suffered from intestinal obstruction whom I introduced in chapter 8. I was really interested in all the deaths she'd had in her life recently, so I started asking her about her grief process. Losing five family members and close friends in twelve months was a big deal. Anyone who had been through that would be grieving. So when she said, "Of course," in response to my question as to whether she had grieved, I wanted to know what grieving meant to her.

"Well," she said, "I've felt really sad about it." Yet I could tell that wasn't enough. I sat there, present and listening. Theresa was silent for a good long while.

"I haven't cried, though," she said. For the first time, she looked at me directly. I had a sense that she was assessing me to see whether I was safe. I held my gaze steady and tried to reassure her that I was safe and could hold the space she needed.

Still, we sat. Silently, I signaled that we had all the time in the world.

Suddenly, a lumbering sound built in her belly. It rose up through her throat. It entered her mouth, and I saw a look of panic. Then the sob fully erupted from her mouth, almost as if she were vomiting. I reached out to hold her, and she accepted my embrace as we sat together. There in my arms, she sobbed and sobbed.

As Theresa cried, I could feel her releasing the sadness stuck inside her. Her entire body began to undulate as the sobs moved through her. Then an uncanny thing happened. She was sad, yes, but I felt her being was flowing with life.

Over time, she began to settle down. She sat back down in her seat. I offered her a tissue, and she took it. Then she sipped a glass of water for a few minutes, shaking slightly. The room felt both calm and potent, like the strange quiet that comes after an Arizona monsoon. We both knew that something incredible had happened—something that she had desperately needed.

After our appointment, Theresa's chronic obstruction immediately dissipated. It seemed that as soon as her emotional state shifted, her body was able to self-correct. She went home to find that her digestion and elimination had become regular again. It turned out that her tears had needed to move first; then the rest of her body could follow.

This provides a clear example of what happens when we try to stop the flow of life: first we become deeply uncomfortable, and then we start to suffer. Our muscles lock up; our organs stop their healthy functioning; we become sick. We misalign with life, because life is moving and we are focused on sitting still. We sit there staring at the dam blocking the flow of life within us.

And when we stare at that dam, we fail to notice the small trickle forming around it.

Find the trickle. Or at the very least, find the place where the trickle is about to start. Give it your energy. Put all your life force there, in that part of you that is finding a path around the dam. Believe in it; trust it. This is life moving through you. As long as you're alive, your life force is flowing.

As you watch this trickle, it will grow. Your life force will tell you how to grow it. Watch it become a stream. Put your attention there until the dam shakes, cracks, and breaks free. When it does, let gratitude for your life force flow. Let your faith in yourself run through you as your life force strengthens.

What can you do the next time you feel stuck? Let things go and realign with life.

Practice: Letting Go

1. This exercise will work best if you get up and move! Put on some upbeat music and start walking around your house or your neighborhood. Let your body move loosely and freely as you walk—you may even let yourself dance a little.

2. As you move your body, consider something that feels stuck in your life. It could be a friendship, a professional endeavor, an identification, a way of thinking, a resentment, and so on. It could also be something physical, provided you don't substitute this exercise for medical treatment; consider a persistent cough, a patch of dry skin, or chronic pain that you're not able to resolve otherwise. Allow the feeling of stagnation to come over you. Feel the sense of stuckness in your whole body.

3. Then imagine that you could hold this stuck thing in your hand. You may even feel one fist become tight. Hold this tightness. Squeeze your hand.

4. While still moving, hold your hand out in front of you, palm up, with the fingers together. Then drop it down and back, opening your fingers slightly. Let the weight of your arm bring your hand down; let life itself move. As you do so, release the stuckness like flowers to the water. Really let it go. You can think or say words that are meaningful to you: "Kutch par wa nay," "It doesn't matter," or any similar phrase that works for you.

5. Once you've let it go, take a moment to appreciate the flow of life moving through you. This is your life force. Honor and cherish it; it will be with you your whole life.

SECRET III

Love Is the Most Powerful Medicine

Chapter 13

LOVE AND FEAR

Susan, a young elementary school teacher, had been my patient for several years when she was in a terrible car accident. Her back was broken in several places. It seemed some sort of miracle she had survived. In her early thirties, she was beloved by many and had a bright future ahead of her, yet the intensity of the accident threatened to cut it short.

I knew she was in good care with the trauma doctors who were treating her. Yet I also knew that she would need holistic support, so I went to visit her in the hospital. I arrived to find her lying immobilized in a hospital bed, her body confined in a full-body cast. The only parts of her body she could move were her mouth, eyebrows, and eyes. She could speak, she could eat, and she could look around; that was it. She had been told she would not walk again. Her brother, an orthopedic surgeon, had confirmed that and added that the possibility she would ever even sit up in a wheelchair was slim.

When I first walked into the room, I was immediately hit with the sense of helplessness that Susan and her family had about the situation. How could they not feel helpless? My eyes traced the contours of Susan's full-body cast. The plaster started just under her chin and extended down her arms and legs. The room contained flowers, cards, and well wishes from her friends, as well as the class of students she was now unable to teach. Yet any sense of cheer felt contrived. It was undeniable that her condition was dire and her usually bright spirit was suffering.

Looking around the sterile hospital room, I trusted that her medical team was taking care of her physical needs. Western medicine is very good at that, especially when it comes to acute injuries and other emergency situations. Susan's doctors had put her bones in the right place and held them there with plaster, protecting her fragile spine so it could have a chance to heal. Yet I felt unsure about the advice she had been given, which suggested that returning to a fully functional existence was impossible. I was even more concerned that she had heard it from her very own brother, who certainly was sharing the best of his medical knowledge but who had the greatest potential to influence Susan's thoughts. I understood his intention: not to sugarcoat the situation or provide Susan with false hope. Yet I found it hard to believe that there was truly nothing to be done.

Yes, Susan was drastically hurt. Yes, her spine had undergone extreme trauma. Yes, she was in a precarious situation. Yet no, I didn't think it was time to pronounce her unhealable. She was young and vibrant, brimming with life force. How could we channel it toward her healing, even in those desperate circumstances?

I pulled up a chair to her bedside. First I sat quietly with her, feeling her fear and grief without pushing them away. She talked a bit and I listened, making the space safe for her to recount her trauma and terror. I knew she trusted me, so I held her concerns with great love. Like others had, I reminded her how beloved she was and how important her life was to the many people whose lives she had touched.

Then, when the moment was right, I asked, "Is there any way you think I can help you?"

With that simple question, I reminded Susan that she had a role in her own healing. This was my first attempt to bring her out of her fear and back to the love that was waiting for her.

To understand what happened next, we first have to understand the relationship between love and fear. It is likely that very few people reading this will ever be in such a precarious position as Susan was after her accident. Yet many of us have felt what she must have felt in the hospital bed: helpless and terrified. What can we do when it seems that everything is stacked against us? What is the right response when we feel we cannot change anything about our circumstances? How can we act when we feel utterly helpless?

When we receive "bad" news, fear is a natural response. Things aren't going well in the here and now. Not only that, but we often wonder how much worse it's going to get. The fear is understandable, but if we stay in that fear, we can shut out nearly everything that might help us resolve the situation. Fear destroys our sense of reason, making it impossible to see things clearly.

That's why part of our collective life purpose is to learn how to move past fear and into love. When we do this, we not only activate our own juice, we also help others do the same. A fearless person is an inspiration to everyone else around them. I don't mean a daredevil, necessarily—I mean a person who approaches life with an open heart. Such people inspire others because going beyond our fear reconnects us with love.

Medicine often underestimates the power of love. These words are so commonly used that they can even sound a bit hokey: *the power of love.* Love is a tricky thing to describe. I cannot explain it to someone who hasn't experienced it any more than I can explain the color green to a person who was born blind. Yet hopefully you've experienced love in your life, and you've already caught a glimpse of what it can do. I hope you've had the chance to know how love can sweep in and change everything, overpowering anything in its presence. It's not hokey. It's not overstated. Love truly is the greatest medicine the world has ever known. It takes life from a passive state (being alive) to an active state (truly living). That's why my third secret is: *Love is the most powerful medicine.* **Our life force is activated by love.**

Love has an uncommon ability to transform everything it touches.

It transforms labor from drudgery to bliss. It transforms laughter from cruelty to joy. It transforms listening from empty sound to a message we can hear. Things become infinitely possible when love is present.

To work with love, we first have to understand its relationship to fear.

When fear steps in, love steps out—and vice versa. My friend Cecile's young son was afraid of the water. The child had a tendency to inhale water through his nose and had become terrified of bathing and swimming. "The water will go up my nose!" he explained to his mother. "Then I can't breathe!"

Cecile was at a loss for what to do, so she connected with a swimming instructor who specialized in that type of trauma. The swimming instructor fixed the problem in a single session by teaching the child to hum underwater. "It's such a simple philosophy," Cecile mused as she sat across from me on the living room sofa. "As long as he keeps humming, he can't inhale the water. When he's out of air to hum, he knows to come to the surface."

On the one hand, the child was right: when we inhale water, we can't breathe. On the other hand, our breath is what keeps the water out. If we develop a habit of inhaling water, humming is the perfect solution.

This is precisely how love and fear work. Love dispels fear, but it is also blocked by fear. The two are often presented together because they're constantly in a push-pull game with each other. If fear is our habit, practicing love is a wise solution. And that practice will take us far, because love is infinitely stronger than fear—*always*. Just as our bodies are born to breathe air, we are born to love. That's why although it's good to address our fear, it's even better to focus on our love. Any effort we put toward love—truly, any effort at all—will self-perpetuate, bringing joy, health, and well-being into our lives.

Another metaphor may help explain it better. Decades ago, Bill and I took our kids to the Carlsbad Caverns in southern New Mexico. This series of caves runs deep beneath the desert. While the heat blazes above, the cold inside the earth is shocking—uncomfortable, even. And the dark is complete. It is as black as the darkest night down there.

When we visited, our guide thrilled us by asking us to turn off our flashlights. One by one, we clicked them off and let the darkness overtake the space. The darkness made everything else acute—we could hear the sound of our breath, the children giggling nervously, their voices echoing around the massive space.

Then the guide lit a single match. The flame was concentrated within the first inch above his matchstick, yet we gasped in wonder as the glow lit up the whole cave.

Many people have remarked upon the power light has to overcome darkness—Gandhi, Anne Frank, and Martin Luther King, Jr., to name a few. There's a reason so many people use this imagery: it illustrates a remarkable and real phenomenon. As my family and I witnessed, it doesn't take much. No matter how much darkness there is, light overcomes it. Light spreads through the entire space. The darkness can't persist in the presence of something as powerful as that.

When looking at darkness and light or inhaling and exhaling, we can focus on only one or the other in any given moment. That means that throughout our lives, we are fundamentally faced with a choice: Will we direct our attention toward love or toward fear?

Chapter 14

CHOICE

Over the years I have been championing holistic medicine, I've found that the idea of choice is one of the trickiest to explain. It's the idea that there's always something we can do, and this is true even when we face our greatest challenges. At its worst, this sounds like blame. You may think, "I didn't choose to get this diagnosis!" or "My loved one didn't choose to lose their job!"—and you're right. That's absolutely the case. I certainly don't consider myself to be the cause of the many difficult things I experienced in my life. I'm not the cause of the health challenges I've faced, either—rickets, malarial hepatitis, kidney stones, and cancer (twice). The fact that we have choice doesn't mean that the bad things that happen are our fault. But as I faced each of those things, I had an opportunity to choose what I would do and how I would respond. Even when we're lost in the dark, each of us can choose how to forge the path ahead. Seen this way, choice is empowering. It lifts us up; it doesn't drag us down.

To a degree, choice happens automatically. We often end up choosing fear without even meaning to do so. Many people have undergone trauma wherein painful events were out of their control. They don't want to feel blamed for the suffering they experience as a result of that trauma—and indeed, I have no intention of blaming them for it.

Yet there is a degree to which suffering *is* within our control. It's natural to seize up in fear when terrible things happen that we cannot control—but how long we remain seized up is, in fact, somewhat up to us. There are aspects of what we make of our traumas, how we move forward, and what we create in our lives in the years and decades to come that are for us to choose. That includes considering whether we need to go into therapy for the things that happened or process them in some other way. In all cases, we can consciously decide how much focus we're going to put on fear and how much we're going to put on love.

Even as we choose, our automatic reactions are likely to tug at us. Shortly after we moved to Arizona in 1955, Bill met a psychologist and psychotherapist named Milton Erickson at a medical conference. Milton was about twenty years older than we were and shared some of our interest in the area modern medicine hadn't fully explored yet—namely, the role of the unconscious.

The conscious mind contains what we're aware of in any given moment. The subconscious expands the conscious to include that which we can think of, imagine, or remember just by giving it attention. But the unconscious includes everything else: the things we assume, believe, or have forgotten we experienced. It includes the automatic reactions we can't quite explain.

Milton was particularly interested in how hypnosis might be used in a clinical setting to make changes in the unconscious that could affect a patient's day-to-day life. Though the conscious and subconscious could be directed with will, as long as the unconscious remained the same, he believed, any strides made in therapy or psychiatry could have only a limited effect, because people were likely to return to their old patterns of behavior.

Milton and Bill began to host a weekly discussion group on Tuesday nights in our living room. It was one of our first acts of connection in the Arizona medical community. Like us, Milton believed that patients could play an active role in their own healing—in his case, by directing their intention toward their unconscious beliefs and the often painful events that had contributed to them. His philosophies would later be used to form a variety of methodologies, such as family systems theory and neurolinguistic programming, and the professionals who furthered his theories after his death are often called "Ericksonians." Even way back in the beginning of his study, Milton firmly believed that nearly anything that had happened in the past could be healed. The healing process could begin only when the conscious mind was directed toward making a change.

Understanding that we are ultimately the ones who choose helps us locate and direct our life force, because in moments of great fear, we often forget how powerful we are. When we face a health challenge, we forget to say "Hello, beloved body. What do *you* need?" When life offers us loss or uncertainty, we forget to ask "Well, now, what am I going to make of this?" Such questions have a transformative power. They activate our curiosity, which cuts through our fear and dispels the idea that we're helpless. They reconnect us to the life force that is living inside us—a life force that is, essentially, love.

Love has the ability to heal our bodies and our hearts. Just as our bodies are built to heal, our hearts are, too. Many of us know people who have experienced great emotional trauma who have healed, and their stories can provide us inspiration to heal ourselves. I've filled this book with stories like that, and you likely have a few of your own, too.

For instance, consider Dr. Elisabeth Kübler-Ross, whose story I told in chapter 11. Elisabeth was hopping mad at the people in her town who blocked her hospice center and ostracized her from the community—and that was before they shot her llama and burned her house down! She was absolutely the victim, in this case, of a definable crime for which no one was ever held accountable, and she needed help to get through the trauma of what had happened. Yet she allowed herself to say "*Kutch par wa nay*" to what she couldn't control in the situation and move on. That was absolutely a choice. She loved herself and her life, and she was willing to choose them over the fear, anger, and pain she was feeling.

Every one of the stories in this book contains an aspect of choice like that. To turn toward life, we have to understand that we can always choose, in every moment. Each second of our lives provides an opportunity. When we truly accept that, we can access the love that is waiting for us. That's why choice is our very first act of self-love. And all love is based on self-love.

How can we find the courage to choose love in the face of fear? Like Elisabeth's story shows us, we start with self-love.

Chapter 15

THE ROLE OF SELF-LOVE

I suppose self-love was a more revolutionary idea when I started talking about it fifty years ago. Today, it's a more natural part of our collective vocabulary. Yet it's one thing to know the term and another to actually live it.

It's only when we know we are lovable that we become love-able. We can't love anyone else until we believe that we ourselves can be loved. That's why it's the first area for us to work on once we've chosen love over fear. So what holds us back from knowing we are lovable?

In some cases, we're held back by unconscious beliefs. Many of us, myself included, were raised with religious beliefs that confuse self-love and pride. We don't let love in because we somehow think we don't deserve it or that accepting it is somehow immoral. You may have heard the adage "Pride cometh before a fall," which is often misunderstood. Pride that is built through false pretenses, such as thinking we are better or more important than others or that our contribution is more worthy, will surely cause us to fall. But self-love is not pride at all. It is gratitude for the life we have been given. When we refuse to love ourselves, we shut out love from everyone else, too. Receiving love requires us to dismantle these beliefs piece by piece.

Self-love is the basis of all love—all the love we give and all the love we receive. It's crucial. And although most of my patients today say that they understand it, when I start questioning them, it becomes clear that deep down, many of them aren't actually sure whether they're worthy of their own love. Many people hold unconscious beliefs based on past experiences that override their conscious thought. That's precisely why we need to consciously direct love back toward ourselves.

Take a moment to ask yourself: *Do I actually believe I'm worthy of the love I give others? Do I believe my body, with all its imperfections, is worthy of love? Do I believe my soul is worthy of love, even though I've made many mistakes in my lifetime? Do I respect myself, admire myself, honor myself, trust in myself?*

If your answer wasn't as strong as you expected it to be, there is no need to fear. It's never too late to work on it. I've spent my whole life learning self-love. I'm getting better at it all the time. Every time something difficult comes my way, I have an opportunity to strengthen self-love through practice. And I had another opportunity to practice it in my nineties when I was diagnosed with breast cancer.

I had faced cancer before, in 1961. Back then, Bill and I had just begun gaining notoriety for our work with holistic health when an egg-shaped tumor began to grow on my thyroid. Within weeks of my first noticing it, it had grown to an inch long. My oldest child was a teenager, and my youngest was just a year old. I was unsure whether to pursue allopathic treatment or try to heal it naturally, so I asked for a dream to tell me what to do.

Right away, I dreamed of the plants that could help me: aloe, ocotillo, and the ash from the burnt wood of aspen trees. I was blessed to have a strong support network at the time, so I cut back on my busy schedule and began an intensive fasting regimen supported by meditation and prayer. I treated myself daily with the plants from my dreams. Over the course of several months, the tumor shrank, and eventually it disappeared.

My decision to heal my tumor naturally spread through the burgeoning holistic health community. People marveled at the miracle that had taken place. As both a leader in natural health and an MD, I thought that it was important that I had demonstrated what is possible.

When I found a tumor in my breast five decades later, I wondered whether I should attempt to heal it that way again. Yet my life had changed drastically since that time. My body was much older. The intensive fasting I had done before would have been harder for it to withstand. At the same time, Western treatments had developed significantly—particularly for the type of tumor I had. I had options that, though still invasive, were much more gentle and better targeted. Most important, I was hard at work on many other projects that were using my life force and giving me juice in return.

Though I wasn't closed to the idea of healing the tumor naturally, I knew it would take a good deal of effort. I didn't feel the same call to go public with my healing and share the miracle with others; it felt much more personal this time. I wasn't terribly afraid, but I was aware that the more quickly I decided, the better my chance of success would be. I asked for guidance and saw that my contemplations and dreams backed up my suspicions: at that point in time, and with that particular tumor, a Western approach was the right choice for me.

That didn't mean I was off the hook for participating in my healing, though. I teamed up with an oncologist and a surgeon. Together, we worked to remove the tumor. They were in charge of radiology and a lumpectomy. I was in charge of visualizing and loving myself into health.

I thought back to what I'd once told a patient about surgery: "When a gardener prunes a tree, he takes away the parts that are no longer adding to the life of the tree. They fulfilled their purpose, and now they're done." My tumor was the same. I loved myself, my body, and my life too much to let it take any more of my life force. Just as I'd done in my first bout with cancer, I put all my focus on that love and refused to let myself fall into fear.

In the weeks before the surgery, I started talking to the lump. I pictured it like a pretty little hand-tooled suitcase. "Darling, we're going to have a family reunion," I told my tumor. "If there are other cancer cells in my body, call them together, and tell them to get in the suitcase and come on the trip." When the time came, I went into the surgery joyfully, knowing that my body would be healthier with that piece removed. I took a similar approach to radiation, choosing to look at it in a matter-of-fact way, like clipping my toenails—there were cells I didn't need anymore, and I was doing what I needed to do to get rid of them. I wasn't mad at the cells or afraid of them, but they were not serving my well-being.

The treatment worked, and my second journey with cancer was as short as my first. I have no doubt that the allopathic treatments I chose were an important step to healing. I'm also certain that the way I thought about receiving those treatments, and the visualization of the suitcase, were just as important. I made the decision with love and supported it with more love. Sure, there was fear, but I refused to feed it. I also refused to reject my body for a few multiplying cells. I felt as proud of my body then as I do today. This body is amazing! I love all the things that it has done and all the things it has yet to do.

Whenever my patients or loved ones are faced with a challenging diagnosis like this, I encourage them to keep on loving their bodies anyway. I also encourage them to visualize their healing, creating their own imagery, like my hand-tooled suitcase.

Some people find creating their own imagery difficult. They want me to come up with an image for them or suggest a right way to do it. It requires a good deal of trust to believe that the image we find will work, and those who are really limited in self-love often struggle to trust themselves, too. But you are the only one who can come up with your imagery; you must find the physician within, the one who knows how to heal, and start to trust.

This is part of how we direct our conscious mind toward transforming the unconscious. The unconscious offers up the images we need to heal. Each of us has to find an image that works for us and feels real, and we have to do it with as pure a love as we can muster. I've seen this age-old method work time and again—even, and perhaps *especially*, when a patient feels skeptical about his or her ability to find the right image. That's precisely when we need to let the unconscious show us how to heal.

Though the ideas about affirmation and visualization are not new, the science that backs it up is still emerging. Yet we are slowly but surely realizing that the relationship between our thoughts and our bodies can be measured. As the Nobel Prize winner Elizabeth Blackburn, PhD, and her colleague Elissa Epel, PhD, found, telomeres (the endcaps on our chromosomes) are affected by thought.[10] That means that although positive thinking doesn't affect our DNA directly, it does affect the way our genes express themselves, which can have profound effects on both our health and our experience of being alive.

Imagery concentrates our thoughts and makes them real in our bodies. As new research emerges around stem cells, which I see as science's answer to the creative life force, it appears that they are affected by how and what we think. Studies are affirming what holistic, spiritual, and often Indigenous healers have been saying for centuries: there's power in recognizing our own role in the healing process because our minds affect everything, right down to the cellular level.

The cells of our body know their jobs. They want to support us by doing what they're here to do. As living human beings, we set our intention; then our cells ally with us to manifest it. It's our job to juice them up with life force, but from that point forward they are participants in everything that happens. The form of medicine I practice, which I call *living medicine*, takes the idea of holistic medicine beyond the medical practitioner. It's a collaborative model between healer and patient that uses therapeutic modalities to enhance and strengthen the life force within a person. The modalities help the healing to take place, but it's important to note that they don't do the healing, they merely direct it. In living medicine, *our own bodies* are actually the driving force in our well-being—and the body naturally includes the mind. Our role is to trust that and to give our cells the love they need to thrive. This is true self-love.

To offer ourselves this type of care, we must become adept at both giving and receiving love. Yet for many people, loving is one thing and letting love in is quite another.

Chapter 16

HOW TO LET LOVE IN

Oftentimes, we undergo challenges that we interpret to mean we are unworthy of receiving love. People leave us, hurt us, or are unable to give us the love we deserve. Painful experiences such as abuse, neglect, and indifference can shape who we become. They leave an imprint on our unconscious that can have massive effects on our health and happiness.

Receiving love can bring up a lot of fear, especially when we've been hurt in the past. That's precisely why we need to focus on it. As hard as it is to get through the fear, doing so will help us receive more love.

One patient, Pamela, struggled to understand that she was lovable. By the time she came to see me in her sixties, she had many physical problems. As I counseled her, it became clear that she simply did not believe she was lovable. Though she was a wonderful school counselor who had helped many troubled children, she couldn't see her value in life. She consistently compared herself to other people and found herself coming up short. It seemed to me that, deep down, she believed herself to be unworthy of life force—perhaps even of life itself.

After we talked about it for a while, I told Pamela what I thought was at the heart of her problems. "It seems to me that you don't believe you can be loved," I said. "Do you have any sense of why that may be the case?"

Pamela laughed. "Now you sound like my mother!" she said. The response shocked me—what on earth had her mother said to her? I asked Pamela what she meant.

"Oh. Well, my mother simply couldn't love me when I was young because I was such an ugly baby. She *wanted* to love me, but it was just too embarrassing," she explained. She told me that she had been born prematurely, which had made her body quite skinny. When she was a child, her mother had told her many times that when friends came over to see the new baby, she would cover Pamela with a towel so only her face was visible. "That way they wouldn't see how ugly you were," her mother would explain. That was compounded by the fact that two years after she was born, her mother gave birth to a healthy baby boy. The long-standing family "joke" was that Pamela was an ugly baby and her brother was a beautiful baby, so obviously, it was easier for her mother to love her brother.

As she spoke, Pamela realized what was already clear to me: it hadn't been a joke. It was a heartbreaking thing that her mother had told her over and over, and it had affected her deeply. She now realized why her self-esteem was so low and why she was so insistent on comparing herself to others, despite how much it hurt her. We ended the session with a big, long hug, during which I tried to give Pamela every drop of the love she had always deserved.

In subsequent sessions, we stopped focusing on Pamela's symptoms and started looking at her lovability instead. First, Pamela learned to let my love in. Then she began to accept the love from her students and their parents, all of whom adored her. Finally, she was able to start loving herself, and the majority of her symptoms evaporated.

Pamela had struggled to receive love from infancy. That may seem young, but our beliefs about ourselves and our worth can form even earlier than that. I want people to know that they are lovable every minute of their lives. That's why I spent so much of my career focusing on loving birth.

In 1969, I attended a talk given by a well-known psychic medium in the United Kingdom. He drew diagrams as he talked, demonstrating the auras he saw around people. Though I do not see auras, I'm nearly always open to hear others' experiences of the world, so I just sat there listening quietly.

Over time I noticed that there were two general types of auras in his pictures: some were contained, swirling around the heads and going back down again, while others became tangled masses above the heads. I asked him about it, and he explained that some people's souls were "tucked in" when they were born, yielding a more cohesive aura, while other people's souls were not, so their auras became twisted and tangled.

The image of the auras he drew has never left me, nor has the idea of being "tucked in." I immediately connected his statement to the loving births I had been facilitating and went on to facilitate for decades to come. I have now attended the births of thousands of babies—sometimes two or three generations in a family. As I receive child after child in my hands, the vast majority of them headfirst, I welcome them to the world with loving presence, assuring them that this plane is safe and gentle and that their soul's return was divinely intended. I hold their precious heads in my hands with reverence. I thank them for their arrival. As I do, I feel I can hear the angels singing.

I invite you to stop reading and imagine for a moment your own birth. Imagine how vulnerable and perfect you were. Imagine how you opened your small eyes with wonder and first beheld the world.

If you'd like, imagine the angels singing.

Hear the swell of their song.

See your infant self bathed in golden light, welcomed to this place.

I ask you to do this small exercise because in order to access self-love, it's essential for us to understand the miraculous nature of our own incarnation.

Consider the details: you, exactly you, formed a body inside your mother and were born into this world. You came here for a purpose, to this exact biological mother and father, whose DNA combined to form your own. Your soul's journey was shaped by the person or people who raised you, whether it was that mother and father, one or the other, or someone else entirely. While you are here, you will change the world, at least in small ways. You will connect with others and help form their lives. You will create beauty. You will give your gifts and share your experiences. Your impact, no matter how large or how tiny, will ripple outward in ways you may never truly understand.

It doesn't matter whether you believe that your life was intended by some creative force or the result of a long chain of random events. Either way, it's marvelous.

When we align with life, the energy of love flows freely into our hearts. Yet many of us are hurt in our lives—either at the moment of our births, if our souls were not tucked in properly, or later on. Shying away from love is a reaction to that pain. But it can be healed.

In fact, you are the one who can heal it. Though others can assist, they can't do it without your participation. Your choice to heal your hurts, to tuck your own soul in, to marvel at your own incarnation is pivotal. It's the match in the cave. It's what begins to overcome the fear that tells you lies about your own worth, and it has the power to set you free.

Sometimes people find it so hard to receive love from humans that it's easier to start with animals. This makes sense to me; animals have fewer opinions and are far less likely to offend us. I've seen many patients begin to let love in through the love of a dog, a cat, or even a horse. I've had numerous dogs over the years, and I thought it was particularly important for my children to have them when they were small. Animals offer unconditional love and are easy for many of us to adore. They remind us that we are lovable and love-able, even when we've forgotten.

Once you're able to receive love, health and happiness will follow. Then the only natural response is to start spreading it to everyone you meet.

Chapter 17

GIVING LOVE TO OTHERS

As a child, I received a strong education in giving love. My parents loved us well, and I credit them with teaching me to receive love by showing me my individual worth. That was part of their greater goal in life: to heal through the power of love.

My parents were devout Presbyterians who understood Jesus' message to be all about love. Today, I realize that people have interpreted (and misinterpreted) Christianity in a variety of ways. When truly aligned with ideals of charity and healing, missionary work is a beautiful thing, but it has also been used in ways that caused harm. Anything can be used or misused; religion is no exception. In the case of my parents, I truly believe that they used their faith rightfully. The basis of it was their commitment to love.

One evening, back in our home after some months in the field, my mother was working at her typewriter. She spent hours with that heavy contraption, lugging it from camp to camp. Like me, my father struggled with reading and writing, so my mother had taken on the task of sending letters back to the Presbyterian mission to account for the work they were carrying out with church funds. That evening, instead of the regular flurry of keystrokes, I heard her start and stop many times. Finally, my father knocked on the door of the study. She indicated that he could enter, and as he did, he left the door ajar just enough for me to overhear their conversation.

My mother sighed as she noted their low conversion rate. Part of their work was to convert the local people, who were mostly Hindu, to Christianity and to baptize them. Yet my parents never focused on that piece of the work; it wasn't where they put their energy.

My father responded by listing some of their most recent accomplishments in healing wounds and curing illnesses, reminding my mother of the important work they were doing. They treated many people who had never received medical care in their lives. They walked right into the leper colonies; they offered touch to those who had been told they were untouchable.

They did so because they were called to spread their own version of the Gospel. Touch was fundamental in their understanding of medicine, as it is in mine. They healed with their love and their hands, just as their beloved Bible stories said that Jesus had done.

Next to the study door, I listened as my father counseled my mother, naming a few of the wonderful people they had helped over the course of the last month and recounting their ailments: extracting a painfully rotten tooth, resetting a poorly healed bone, treating a child's infection. "We're doing the work, Beth," he said.

"I suppose that's so," my mother mused. "We may not have the numbers, but we're doing the work."

My parents spent the majority of their years serving patients in India, and they both lived long, happy, fully juiced lives. In fact, it was hard even to mourn their deaths, because their very lives had felt like a celebration. I missed them, but I wasn't sad for them. In fully loving, they had fully lived.

The way my parents treated their patients had an important influence on me—not only in my medical career but in the way I have always treated human beings my entire life. They taught me to love *absolutely everyone.*

Now, I want to be clear that loving everyone doesn't mean that we have to agree with everyone. It doesn't mean that we approve of everything everyone does or that we necessarily want to spend a lot of time with them. *Loving* is an energy that goes beyond *liking*. There were plenty of patients whom I struggled to like, and I'm sure the same was true of my parents with the patients they treated. But if I can't love someone, I consider it my problem, not the other person's, so I'd find a way to love them anyway. I'd work to find any small thing I had in common with them—maybe we both loved our kids, or we both enjoyed the desert landscape. If I couldn't find that, I'd look for anything I liked about them, no matter how trivial—perhaps I liked their hairdo or the way they hugged. I've found time and again that my love wants to grow; I just need to build it a trellis it can grow along. Loving is just letting the energy flow into and out of the heart freely, without stopping it. Seen this way, loving is a key part of our health and well-being. It's essential.

Even when we understand this, life can always throw us something unexpected that shakes us to our core. In such moments fear can grab hold of us, even if we're well versed in love. Once we get love flowing both into and out of our hearts, how do we resist the temptation to fall back into fear?

Chapter 18

LOVE AND MIRACLES

Perhaps you've been working on love for a good long while, and you've already made progress in your ability to give and receive it. Then something unexpected happens: you're demoted, your company goes belly up, a relationship crumbles, or someone gets sick. Part of using love as medicine means searching for love even—or perhaps especially—in those dark times.

Here is a scenario I have seen many times over as a doctor: a patient's health gets out of balance, he or she locks up in fear, then he or she turns away from his or her physical body by disconnecting from it or making it into an enemy. This is especially true when we feel as though our body has betrayed or is about to betray us.

One of my patients, Carolyn, had been struggling to get pregnant. Conception didn't come easily to her, carrying a pregnancy to term even less. Despite our best efforts to help her have a baby, she had suffered five miscarriages, all of which occurred around the same point in gestation.

She became pregnant for a sixth time and was cautiously optimistic. Things seemed to be progressing normally, but then she started bleeding right at the same point at which she'd miscarried before.

She called me in a panic. Her fear was strong, and she didn't know what to do. "I'm just certain I'm going to lose this baby," she sobbed. "I feel so helpless, as if there's nothing I can do to stop it."

I didn't know whether I could save her baby, but I felt certain that if she couldn't decrease her fear, she needed to increase her love.

"What your baby needs most right now is your love," I told her, "and that's true whether the child lives or dies." Of course, I couldn't tell Carolyn not to be afraid—she was naturally terrified. But I could bring her focus back to love.

I told her to put a castor oil pack onto her abdomen and have a conversation with her baby's soul, telling it how much she wanted to bring it into the world and pleading with it to stay. "Talk to your child," I said. "You're in this one together."

Carolyn spent the evening speaking to her child. She explained why she and her husband wanted to have a baby and how much they already loved the body that was forming in her womb. She pleaded with the child's soul to stay but remained firm that she would accept whatever was decided—that she wouldn't stop loving her baby, no matter what.

By the next morning, she had stopped bleeding. She came in for an ultrasound, and I checked for cardiac activity. The baby was alive.

As the months went on, Carolyn's pregnancy seemed to be progressing without problems. Her son came to full term, and I was blessed to attend his birth. Once again, I heard the angels singing. But as I held his face in my hand, I gasped.

He had the scar from a cleft lip and palate that we called a "harelip" at the time. This is a serious condition that can take many surgeries to correct. I'd never seen one heal on its own, but this one appeared to have done precisely that. I smiled down at Carolyn, remembering the night she'd conversed with her child. "The great surgeon was at work!" I exclaimed, handing her a perfect baby boy.

Later, I went back and looked up the stages of fetal development to refresh my memory. The moment when Carolyn had bled and prayed with her child was the exact time when the soft palate is formed. I had every reason to believe that she had not only loved herself into healing but helped her son in utero heal, too.

I firmly believe that the fact that Carolyn gave her son love kept him alive. She did so by turning away from the darkness of her fear, despite the high stakes, and reconnecting with the strongest light available to her—in this case, the love she had for her child.

I've seen many other patients do the same. Several years ago, my friend Evelyn was preparing to walk a long section of the Camino de Santiago pilgrimage trail. It had been a lifelong dream for her, and she had long imagined how she would go from village to village, sleeping in guesthouses and eating simple food in the Spanish countryside.

Then she suddenly suffered a knee injury that left her barely walking. She came to see me in a panic.

"Dr. Gladys, what if I'm not able to take this trip?" she asked. "I've been planning it for years. We'll be walking miles and miles every day on an uneven path. I need my knee to be strong, and I don't know how it will ever heal in time!"

"Tell your knee what you need it to do and why," I advised her. "Then love it into health. Talk to your stem cells. Strengthen them with your love and faith." Evelyn spent the next several months praying and meditating for her knee to heal for one express purpose: for her to complete the spiritual mission she had dreamed of for years.

Now, we'll never know if that was what healed her knee or not. We'll never know how things would have gone had she not prayed. But we *do* know that she walked the section of the trail she had always intended to walk, not only with a pain-free and functioning knee but with a renewed dedication to her goal. Her contemplation made the trip even more meaningful because before she even started, she completed an exercise in great faith.

The truth about life is that there are many things we don't know. We don't know, when we receive bad news, how we will find a silver lining. But even just believing has power. It marks the moment we choose, catapulting us out of fear and into love. This alone may heal what ails us. Even when it doesn't, it's bound to bring our lives increased meaning and happiness.

Choosing love in the face of great fear is, in fact, a miracle all on its own. Yet sometimes it creates other types of miracles, too.

Susan, whose tragic car accident I shared in chapter 13, experienced this. As I sat at her bedside, I held her fear and tenderly offered her a choice: What was she going to do in this seemingly impossible circumstance? I knew she had to come up with her own visualization, one that would work for her, just like my hand-tooled suitcase when I had breast cancer. It had to be totally real for her, and it had to be based in love.

I started by explaining to her how bones heal. I told her about osteoblasts, which build connections between bone cells, and osteoclasts, which break them down. I explained the role of peptides and the fact that bones know how to heal themselves if given the chance. "Your body *can* heal," I assured her. "It may not be easy, but it's possible. Choose to see your beautiful body as healthy and strong."

Susan's accident occurred not long after Hurricane Katrina hit New Orleans, and stories of the plans to rebuild were all over the news. As she lay there immobilized, Susan found herself thinking about New Orleans a lot. She could see it being built day after day. Her mind was left with nothing else to do, so she imagined roads being laid and buildings being built. At first, she explained that she didn't know why that visualization came to her; she didn't connect it to our conversation. It seemed to her to be only a strange obsession that arose from her boredom.

Over time, the doctors began to report that unexpected things were happening. Somehow, Susan's spine was beginning to heal in ways they hadn't imagined.

Susan realized that her strange obsession was actually a visualization. She increased her practice, understanding that the "city" she was building in her mind was in fact the bony tissue in her spine. She watched as the workers built buildings and bridges—her osteoblasts. She oversaw wheelbarrow after wheelbarrow of debris removed—her osteoclasts. Over time, her medical team removed the cast. She was able to sit up, then move to a wheelchair.

Just over a year after her accident, she began to walk again.

In living medicine, we are constantly working to give and receive love. We find a way to let this pursuit give us juice. When we make loving a part of our everyday existence, we perpetuate life.

This happens on a large scale as we accept more and more love from the world, allow it to land in our hearts, and begin radiating it outward to the people around us. It also happens on a small scale, as we learn to love every part of our being. The nourishment we give ourselves matters, right down to our cells—and we don't need to wait until we're suffering to start offering ourselves love as medicine.

Practice: Loving Yourself into Healing

1. First get quiet, and then allow a complaint to rise to the surface. It could be something physical—an ongoing medical issue, a short-term injury—or even something emotional, such as a relationship that isn't working out.

2. Consider your complaint, and wait until an image emerges to encapsulate it. Don't overthink this; just let whatever comes come. The image may be moving or still. It may be a thing, a place, even a person. Once you have your image, take a moment to really look at it. What shapes, colors, and textures arise?

3. Ask the image: *What do you have to show me? What do you need?* Is it offering information about your physical health, your mental health, your soul's journey, your relationships? In some way, your mind has offered you this image to show you something. What is it? You may find one answer, or you may find more than one.

4. See your image wrapped in love, held in the unconditional loving embrace of the entire universe. Hear the angels singing once again, just as they did the day you were born. Thank the image and allow it to fade away.

5. Now it's time for a hug. Don't shy away from this, even if you feel a bit silly doing it—it's a transformative practice! Place your hands on opposite shoulders, crossing your arms in front of your heart, and curl your shoulders in. Let your chin drop as you do so, squeezing your hands and giving yourself a good hug. Give yourself as strong a hug as you would give anyone else who needed it.

6. While you're hugging yourself, check in with your heart. Assess where it is today—how lovable, and love-able, do you feel? Receive the answer without judgment. You can repeat this gesture, hugging yourself, anytime you want to assess how love is flowing through you.

SECRET IV

You Are Never
Truly Alone

Chapter 19

LIFE IS CONNECTION

My favorite memories from childhood come from our winter field camps. I loved the sense that everyone had a job to do and that the work was joyful. I loved the idea that we all relied upon one another. I loved knowing that we were far away from others but together, connected. I think fondly about those times; they instilled in me a strong belief in community.

One night, we were gathered around the table in our family tent, playing word games after dinner, when Ayah popped in. "Sadhu is here," she said, smiling. Hindu sadhus were a common sight in India, but less common in our camp, and I knew exactly which sadhu she was talking about. All five of us children jumped to our feet—Gordon was so small, he might not have even known why he was jumping—and ran outside, our parents following behind.

He was a tall man with dark, penetrating eyes that radiated mysticism from way back. Today, I know I was in the presence of a profoundly old soul, though such talk would have been blasphemous to me at the time. Sadhu Sundar Singh was a Christian convert who refused the Anglicization of Christianity. He believed that the best way to spread his faith around India was simply to act as Jesus had acted and to remain fully Indian while doing so. He dressed in the faded saffron *dhoti* of a sadhu, wrapped his head in a turban, and kept a full beard. He smiled when he saw us. "I've missed you, children," he said.

Sadhu Sundar Singh came to visit our camp every winter after spending his summers in Tibet. He always traveled by foot, and he'd spend a week or two at our camp, eating good meals and delighting the camp children with songs and stories. People naturally gravitated toward him; his very presence facilitated connection. I emulated that and knew that when I grew up, I wanted to bring others toward me, too. I wanted to shower my love upon children as he did, to bring hope to everyone who met me, and to tell my stories joyfully to anyone who cared to listen. I wanted to live my truth through connecting with others.

On a fundamental level, we're all connected. It's easy to forget this and see ourselves as separate beings. After all, I'm me, wrapped in my own skin, and there you are, wrapped in yours. Yet we are social creatures, and we depend on one another to survive. No matter how hard we may try to separate ourselves, we are part of a community, for better or worse. We're part of a family, a culture, a country, a continent, a species. We connect through shared experiences and shared genes. We literally share the air we breathe.

We may be separate beings, but we're one community. We have a collective life force. Just as our individual life force requires tending, this collective life force does, too.

I was first struck by this idea in 1969 when Bill and I traveled to Israel and toured a kibbutz. That night, we stayed up late buzzing with energy, discussing what we'd seen—how everything in the community was interconnected. Everybody had a purpose, everybody had a job. What the kids were doing in school had to do with what was happening on the farm, in the clinic, or in the kitchen. Everyone was both contributing to and receiving from the collective life force.

That trip was part of the inspiration for the Baby Buggy program that I ran with nurse-midwife Barbara Brown throughout the 1970s and 1980s. The program encouraged supported home births, where women could be attended by their loved ones as well as trained professionals in the comfort of their home. Our specially outfitted van would park in the driveway of a laboring woman while we monitored her progress. If intervention or a medical transport was required, we had everything we needed. In most cases, the Baby Buggy just stayed there, parked, while women gave birth to healthy, happy babies in their own homes. In some cases, we used it to transport the mother, the baby, or both to the hospital. In all cases, our van with its giant stork painted on the side sent a clear message to the community: A new soul is arriving! Welcome it!

A true sense of community seems rare in our modern age. Even before the pandemic, many media reports were noting that we are experiencing a crisis of loneliness. Loneliness has been identified as a problem in numerous countries and across a range of demographics.[11] This sense of disconnection wreaks havoc on the body. One study at Brigham Young University showed that feeling lonely has the same effect on longevity as smoking fifteen cigarettes a day.[12] Poor social relationships have been associated with a 29 percent increase in the risk of heart disease and a 32 percent increase in risk of stroke.[13]

At the same time, the data show that positive social connections help us thrive. The author Ashton Applewhite has noted that social connection is a main indicator of happy and healthy aging. She also recommends multigenerational friendships, an idea that is echoed by numerous studies showing the positive effects being around small children has on older people facing questions of purpose.[14] While marriage in general is associated with decreased risk of cardiovascular disease, troubled marriages are associated with increased risk.[15] According to the Harvard Study of Adult Development, the quality of our relationships at age fifty is the greatest predictor of our health and well-being at age eighty.[16]

Life comes from our connection, is supported by our connection, and creates connection. We are happiest and healthiest when we are contributing to and drawing from our collective life force. This idea is the basis of my fourth secret for you: *You are never truly alone.* **Connecting with community amplifies our individual life force by realigning it with the collective life force.**

This means that we thrive when we receive others' attempts to connect with us. And since connection is something we offer as well as accept, we are the ones who determine the health of our communities. Each of us is responsible for creating a supportive network for ourselves. In doing so, we contribute to the overall network that supports others. Our giving doesn't even have to be altruistic because it's self-serving. As my son Bob said when he was a child, "Hey, Mom, I think I've figured it out! If I make a friend and he makes a friend and he makes a friend, it will go all the way around the world and come back to me!"

I've seen thriving communities all over this globe. I've noticed the greatest sense of community joy in groups of people who are working together, even—or perhaps especially—in the face of great struggles. It doesn't take perfect people or a lot of money to help a group thrive; it takes working with what we have and finding a way for that to be enough.

I was raised to believe in the power of connection. I came from a strong family and a vibrant community in which people helped one another and were connected. I continue to create a thriving family, despite the many things we've been through, and have always been greatly involved in the world around me. I prioritize my social relationships because I know how it feels through my whole being when I'm giving to and receiving from others.

I suspect you know what that feels like, too. I hope that at least once in your life, you have felt what it's like to be completely supported. I hope that you've had the chance to support someone else for a moment and you've felt that sense of connection. If you have, you may remember how it energized you. You may recall how renewed life force moved through you, propelling you forward. The increase of that life force indicates the importance of community.

For decades I have held steady on a single dream: a Village for Living Medicine, in which healing, living, and learning will be rolled into one. In some ways, my vision is based on the traveling camps of my childhood. In others, it's a whole new paradigm, where people would come to live and work together to heal. We are social beings; we are meant to be together. This is how we thrive.

Though many of us know this on an intellectual level, it's becoming harder and harder to put into practice. The United States (as well as much of the world) is splitting down ideological lines. Family members are unable to connect with one another, opting to spend holidays and celebratory events in their separate corners. More and more marriages end in divorce. Our houses and yards get bigger as we retreat into our individual electronic devices. The more we have, the more we spend time apart. Even if we *want* to connect, at least theoretically, it feels as if it's too hard to get our needs met. Perhaps we've even forgotten how to do so.

As I watch this happen around me, I can't help but wonder: If we enjoy connection and know it's good for us, why do we avoid it?

Chapter 20

EMBRACING IMPERFECTION

When my first child, Carl, was born, I was living in Cincinnati and had made friends with another young mother down the road who had a son the same age. We were both interns at the same hospital, and we had some things in common. Carl and Harry started playing together as soon as they were old enough to be off our laps. They got along, but each played in a different way—in part because our parenting styles were so different. Carl was an adventurous kid whom Bill and I encouraged to crawl, climb, and get dirty. Harry's mother sent him out to play wearing gloves and sometimes on a leash.

Nowadays, there's plenty of information available that tells young parents the importance of letting their kids get a little dirty. Most people know that an overly sterile environment isn't great for their children's development. But Harry's mother's medical training had focused on germ theory, which was solely about killing diseases, and she was doing the best she could with the information she had. Like so many other women, she had been taught that there were specific things she could do to be a "good mom," and keeping her son away from germs was one of them.

Both Harry and his mother were also my patients. I saw them a lot because Harry was frequently sick. He picked up all sorts of bugs, despite his mother's best efforts. Once, as Carl was playing in the dirt while Harry sat quietly watching, she asked me, "Why is it that Carl is only rarely sick but Harry comes to see you in the clinic so often? I'm so careful with him!"

I laughed and explained that Carl likely had a stronger immune system. I exposed him to the world, and he was more resilient for it.

This story isn't remarkable on its own. Yet when taken as a metaphor, it has a lot to teach us. There are some things that are truly harmful—hot stoves, high cliffs, venomous snakes—and Harry's mother would have been right to protect him from those. But she took it too far, and he suffered as a result. This is precisely how community works. Yes, some people can truly hurt us, it's true. But when we overly protect ourselves from others, we cut ourselves off from the very interactions that could serve us. We were born in a world full of people because we're meant to be around people, with all the messiness that entails.

We often don't interact with one another because we don't want to get our hands dirty. We don't want to deal with what we perceive to be others' deficits. We want to protect ourselves so we can't be disappointed. But in the process, we miss out on life.

The advent of modern conveniences has made this easier. We have essentially sterilized our lives of the discomfort of "needing" one another. Today, if we are sufficiently economically comfortable, we've set up the entire world so we don't have to ask anyone for anything. Apps, instead of neighbors, help us pick up our car from the mechanic or get a ride to a doctor's appointment. On a busy school night, dinner can be ordered in minutes via delivery. We can hire people to walk our dogs, assemble our furniture, and wash our cars with the click of a button. The more we progress, the more it seems that we simply want the convenience of not having to ask anything of our neighbors and friends. We're constructing a community-for-hire.

Gone are the days of borrowing a cup of sugar, let alone raising a barn with neighbors.

Perhaps I sound like an old lady complaining about how the world is changing. Yet I'm pointing toward something much bigger here: We need to borrow cups of sugar. We benefit from barn raising. Living together in this way forces us to connect, even in small ways. In the past, our messy, frequent interactions made sure we knew our neighbors and understood what was happening in one another's lives. They kept us vital by providing a safeguard against isolation.

Modern life increasingly allows us to reduce the interactions required for day-to-day living, supporting this effort with the idea that we're happiest if we interact with others only when we want to do so. Yet reducing our interactions is so costly. We lose so much when we don't connect with community. We miss out on a fundamental piece of being human.

Choosing community does have its trade-offs. For one thing, it's certainly less controlled. I saw that in 1958, when Bill and I moved into our second home in Arizona. It was a large adobe house that was nearly indestructible—perfect for our busy family of seven, which quickly became eight. We ate dinner together every evening, and we usually had upward of fifteen people around our big oak dining table. We didn't worry about keeping the house neat or making the food perfect. The whole point was to be together.

People came and went from that house so often that one time, when a series of neighborhood burglaries brought a policeman to our door to warn us about locking up at night, we realized that though all eight of us lived there, not one of us had a key. In those years, my husband and I frequently hosted fundraisers for the various organizations we founded and supported. We also hosted talks by a series of medical professionals and healers from a wide range of backgrounds, most of whom stayed a few days for less formal discussions around the table. And nearly every day, we welcomed a raucous houseful of children from the neighborhood.

When considering what we valued as parents, Bill and I chose to make our home a place where kids and adults alike could come to have fun and be themselves. In doing so, we gave up the option of having a calm, quiet, or spotless house. It may have led to some chaotic years, but I have no regrets. Creating community requires allowing a little chaos.

One afternoon I found a moment to relax in the bathtub, letting the stress of motherhood and work release from me. Our bathroom had two doors, one going into a bedroom and one into Bill's study. Just as I was closing my eyes and relaxing into the water, the door to the bedroom popped open. A wild-eyed boy ran into the bathroom, passed straight by the sink, and flung open the door to the study beyond. No sooner was he through the door than a little girl came running behind him and followed him back out into the study. Then the next ones came: a bigger one made three, then a shaggy-headed one made four, then a tiny impish one, five. In just a few moments, ten kids ran into the bathroom, past me in the tub, and out the other door. Only three of them were mine, and none of them even noticed I was there. Part of me was annoyed—there I was, stark naked in the tub, trying to get a moment to myself. The other part of me marveled at the joyful and raucous home I'd been able to create for my children.

Accepting others into our lives means that things are going to be somewhat disordered and messy. We can't live in community and expect everything to be perfect or exactly the way we want it to be. Yet there's something so important to be gained from imperfection. I understand the desire for control; each of us is on our own path, and we want to be in charge of how we walk it. But the beauty is that our paths can and will intersect with the paths of others. This can be such a beautiful thing; we can share the way in which we traveled the path, we can tell others what we've learned and where we're going, we can learn from them. From one angle, this could be seen as stressful. But short-lived, acute stress may actually be good for us. That doesn't mean we should spend a lot of time around consistently negative or abusive people—ongoing stress, of course, causes plenty of problems. Yet research suggests that some stress may have positive benefits.[17]

When we try to create a sterile world, devoid of the imperfections and annoyances of human interaction, we work against our own life force and become weaker—just like poor little Harry in his gloves.

Yet we live in a society that tries to convince us that we have to like everything about everyone in order to get along. In such a polarized world, this sort of thought process can make it hard to know who to befriend. If community is so important, how can we start to build it?

Chapter 21

FIND YOUR FRIENDS

As I wrote in chapter 17, I aim to love everyone, but that doesn't necessarily mean I *like* everyone. In the same way, it can help to find a way to be friends with everyone—to varying degrees. When we commit to befriending everyone, we can accept them and have some sort of friendship with them regardless of who they are or what they believe. We can find the friend within them, even if it's only a small slice of who they are.

Elisa, a college student, was home for her winter break when she came in for a bit of eczema on her elbow. Her mother had been my patient for years, so I'd known Elisa since childhood, and though she tended to be anxious, she generally relaxed after a minute or two. But this time her hug felt a little off, as though she wasn't fully present with me, and even after I held her arm to examine it, her adrenals seemed active. Though she was sitting still, her eyes were shifting and her arm trembled just a bit in my hands. Eczema, as those who struggle with it know, is often exacerbated by stress.

"You can put a little castor oil on this and it should clear up, but call if it doesn't and I'll prescribe a steroid," I said. Then I moved my hands down her arm and held her hand instead, squeezing it gently.

"Now, Elisa, what's really going on?" Her hand felt cold in mine, and I hoped to give her some of my warmth.

"Oh, coming home for the break isn't all I thought it would be, that's all, " she said brusquely. "It's fine. I'll just get through the holidays and go back to school."

"What isn't what you thought it would be?" I asked, wondering if something was happening in the family.

She explained that her family was fine, and talking about what was going well seemed to soften her defenses. Then she admitted the truth: "It's just that it's a little weird with my friends. I mean, with my best friend, Chloe. She moved in with her boyfriend, I'm in the dorms—our lives are so different now. Like, I reach out to her, but we don't have anything in common anymore. It feels a bit surface level, you know?"

"I know."

"And I'm just not really that into superficial friendships. They feel like a waste of time and energy. So I don't know if I wasted my time with her or not, or if I'm wasting it now . . . it's just a little hard, I guess."

I smiled at Elisa. Her hand had warmed up a bit; just talking about what was happening had brought her back to life. I told her about some of my dear friends in childhood—the ones whose adult lives connected with mine and those who didn't. I told her about Peter, my lifelong friend who had grown up with me in India, met and married my dear friend Alice in Cincinnati, and ended up as my neighbor in Arizona. "Some friends stay around, others leave and come back. It's true that some dear friendships fade away—but they're all worthy, and they're never a waste. Think of the spring flowers we have here in Arizona," I said, gesturing to the landscape out the window. "Those African daisies, their roots are superficial and they only bloom for a few weeks. But a saguaro's roots go way down—deep enough to withstand high winds and periods of drought. Neither one of these plants is more beautiful than the other. Yet they both help this place come alive. Your friendship with Chloe hasn't ended; it's just changed."

As Elisa and I talked, I explained that some friendships are meant to be deep and span decades. These are the people we depend on when things get difficult. Other friendships are meant to be short. They serve a specific purpose and come to a natural end. Still others, whether they last years or minutes, stay on the surface level. They're friendly and positive, but in relationships like these we never get to know each other more deeply. I know thousands of people, and on some level, I consider all of them friends.

"I consider you a friend, too, you know," I said, and Elisa smiled. "You're younger than me, and since you were a child when I was already grown up, it may seem strange to think about it that way. But I have no idea how old your soul is, and you don't know how old mine is, either. I don't know how we'll know each other in the future. Really, anything is possible—just like with your friend Chloe." I squeezed her hand.

"I thought Chloe and I would be best friends forever . . . and maybe we will. Maybe we won't." Elisa sighed. "I just don't want to be the only one putting effort in."

"It sounds like that's stressful to you," I observed.

"It is. But I think if I stopped trying to make something happen, I'd feel less stressed about it. I'd just let it go where it goes."

"Exactly. You can do your best to reach out to her, but you can't control where this life is going." We talked a little more, and Elisa seemed to relax into the idea. She agreed to reach out to Chloe again while they were both home for the holidays, and then I sent her on her way. She never did contact me about a steroid cream, so I imagine the castor oil (and maybe the talk) worked just fine.

I find a way to be friends with everyone by searching for the friend within them. I find the point—even if it's only one—where our life force flows together, and I lean into it. This may create a long inter-action or a short one; it may be deep or it may be shallow. Regardless, in that interaction, we are friends. We just take it day by day.

To build a stronger community of friends, start with the people in closest proximity to you: your neighbors. Move on to the people you interact with professionally, the people who are friends with your family members, the supermarket checkers and gas station attendants and dentists and tax attorneys and dog groomers in your life. Be friends with children, with teenagers, with older people. Make everyone your friend, even if only in a limited way, and lean into that friendship. All it takes is a little kindness and curiosity. You just have to look for the part of you and the part of them that can be friends and go forward from there.

It's also important to allow the universal flow to push new people your direction. Ask yourself: Who has crossed my path recently? Who needs my attention and my love? When we keep our eyes open to notice who comes our way, who needs us or has something to offer or both, we open ourselves to the universe speaking to us through others.

There's a danger in thinking that we have to agree on everything to enjoy each other's company. This pushes everyone to extremes. It's natural that when someone's life looks like ours, it's easier to find common points of connection. But it's sometimes the people who are most unlike us who push us to see things in a new way. That means there's great meaning in interacting with people we don't like that much. When we approach people who think very differently from us with curiosity instead of condemnation, we grow.

When I first moved to Ohio, I was a fish out of water. The women with just enough stayed home with their kids, and the women with less than that worked, but none of them was as educated as I was and none of them worked by choice. I was used to feeling like the odd one out; I'd gotten through it in college, when it had felt as though I was the only one in Ohio (besides Margaret) who had been raised among elephants and spoke Hindustani, and I'd gotten through it in medical school, where my ideas about healing had put me at odds with the other aspiring doctors around me. I'd spent years in a profession dominated by men, learning over and over how to hold my own. But I still longed for someone like me—and I wasn't finding it in that coal town. Margaret was living two hours away, which was a godsend, and Bill's brother and his wife were close by, too. That kept me going for the first few years.

Beyond that, it seemed that no one took me seriously as a doctor. People often preferred to be treated by Bill or the other male doctors in town. When we started there, we were two of six general practitioners, but one by one they all retired, and then Bill was sent to service out of state. That meant that everyone who had been skeptical of a woman doctor eventually became my patient.

Of course, I showed up with the same knowledge and same love I'd always had, and in short order I won over most of the town. That was when I started experiencing the opposite problem. It was such a close-knit place, and I was so friendly and open, that people had no sense of what was appropriate in a doctor-patient relationship. They'd approach me in the grocery store, in the bank, on the street, always looking for medical advice. One time I tried to go to the movies with my brother-in-law and his wife, and I was paged over the theater's intercom by the police. Someone had a small problem—not an emergency, mind you—and they couldn't find me, so they'd called the police, who'd gotten onto their radios and tracked me down.

Then I got the mumps—a common occurrence back before there was a vaccine—and was hospitalized two towns over for several weeks. I was about as sick as I'd ever been, and I couldn't even take care of the kids, who were all in bed with fever themselves. Yet as I was the only general practitioner around, people just couldn't let me be in the hospital. They'd make the drive up the river to sneak in to ask me about this or that infection or come up to the window and yell up, "Dr. Gladys!" I was really struggling and needed to rest, so eventually Bill and Edith Gilmore, some doctor friends from the hospital, sneaked me back to their house, IV bag and all, and I spent my final days with the mumps recovering secretly in their living room. It was an ironic shift, from being outright rejected to being so needed that I couldn't even heal properly myself.

Though I've always found a way to lighten things with humor, my experience with the mumps highlights a major issue many people face when they try to build community: boundaries. It can be hard to know how to interact with people who don't respect our space or our needs. It's healthy for us to interact with people who are unlike us and even sometimes with people we don't particularly like, but what about those who either actively want to take our life force away or can't keep themselves from doing so? How can we find the friend within everyone and connect, thereby contributing to our common life force, without becoming drained?

Chapter 22

HOW TO SET BOUNDARIES

Setting healthy boundaries starts with knowing who we are and what we came to do. We must first understand what gives us juice and what drains it, because that shows us what's on our soul's path and what's interfering with it. To set and maintain boundaries in just the right place, we have to know ourselves really well. We can look to others who embody this self-assuredness for inspiration, but even then, each of us has to find our own way.

My sister, Margaret, was an important role model throughout my life. In many ways, she took after our mother, walking to the beat of her own drum without needing to put others down for their beat. Margaret's quiet goodness set an example for me. As a child, she gave me something to fight against, but once I learned to stop fighting, I spent the rest of my life emulating her.

When Margaret's first child was born, she and her husband lived in a small home with Mother Courtwright, her mother-in-law, who had a bedroom upstairs. I went to visit when the baby was still in arms. One day, the baby was crying, and it seemed that nothing Margaret did was helping. In retrospect I see that the child was likely gassy or colicky—it had nothing to do with Margaret's care. But Mother

Courtwright came downstairs regardless and immediately started telling Margaret what to do.

Underneath her suggestions was a judgmental, confrontational energy. She seemed to think that Margaret wasn't suited to be a mother. Her tone was negative, almost nasty. I watched as my sister continued to rock and bounce her baby, swaddling her more tightly and holding her close. Eventually, Mother Courtwright finished speaking and went back upstairs.

Margaret continued to hum to her baby softly, completely unperturbed. I was surprised by that because being treated like that would have really frustrated me. I asked my sister how it was possible that she was so unbothered by the incident.

"Oh, she's just like that," Margaret said between coos, her voice bouncing slightly to the beat of her knees. "That's none of my business, though. I don't have energy for it. All my energy is going right here, to my child."

Mother Courtwright lived another twenty years, and she criticized my sister during nearly all of them. But by the time she died, she had come to respect her—so much so that she left Margaret her car in her will.

I have thought about that moment in my sister's living room many times. Her statement "I don't have energy for it" is the clearest expression of boundaries I have ever found. She didn't mean that she didn't possess the energy; she meant that she was choosing to spend it on something else. Family was really important to Margaret, and it felt right to her to have her mother-in-law in her home. This was what it took for her to make it work.

Boundaries are a hot topic in today's culture. Yet we often think of them as ways to keep people out, like fortress walls. I believe this is a misunderstanding. Boundaries come from deep within us; they're about how we choose to spend our energy, what's worth our attention, and what isn't.

In that way, our boundaries are entirely up to us. We often can't control who comes our way or what energy they bring, and putting too much effort into the losing battle of trying to do so drains our life force. But we can always be in charge of how much attention we give the parts of people we don't like. Eventually, if there's very little positive life force to feed, the relationship will become quite surface level or even taper off. Yet there's no need to exclude any *person*, because all we have to exclude is his or her negative energy.

Seen this way, creating good boundaries doesn't require us to keep people out; it requires us to allow the best parts of them in.

One of my patients experienced that when she developed lung cancer. Patty was a longtime smoker, and her condition advanced quickly, so, shortly after her diagnosis, she was hospitalized. I called to check in with the doctors treating her in the hospital, expecting that their efforts would at least be effective enough to get her home.

"She's not doing well," the doctor on the other end of the phone told me. "She's severely anemic, and she's too weak to go home."

"Can you give her a transfusion?" I asked.

"We're trying," the doctor answered, "but she won't let us. Her body may be weak, but she sure is stubborn!"

I went to the hospital to see if I could talk some sense into her. I explained that if she didn't get the transfusion, she would likely die.

"I know," Patty explained, "but it's just not right. I can't let someone else's blood flow in my veins. I don't even know the person. I'm not sure whether I'd even like them. Besides, what if there's some disease in there? It just isn't right. Maybe my body can heal without it."

I heard her concern, but as I looked at her charts, it was clear that she needed the help. Her body *could* heal, but trying to do so with such a low iron level was putting her at an unnecessary disadvantage.

I thought it might help her to reframe it, taking her thoughts away from the idea that she was in a sick body that needed blood and toward something miraculous: that perhaps she was being faced with a sacred opportunity to receive love. I said that it was beautiful that someone in this world loved her enough to give her their lifeblood. It was the very highest and best part of them that offered it, regardless of who they were otherwise. Her body was telling her that she was very weak and that this type of support was necessary. Luckily, someone in the community had donated blood for that very reason. It didn't matter who they were. It mattered only that they had cared enough to help.

That switch in perspective made all the difference. Patty was able to see the donor blood as a gift of love that came from the very best part of the donor. Sure enough, she received the transfusion and she quickly felt much better. Through accepting support from the community, she received the strength she needed to fight her cancer.

Our boundaries are a reflection of who we are and what we need—and since those factors are both in flux, our boundaries are meant to move, too. This doesn't mean we should let other people move them. It means we need to be able to check in with ourselves regularly and know what we need, asking ourselves about the exact shape of our puzzle piece in every moment, and adjust accordingly. Every so often, doing so can even help others find the shape of their own puzzle piece and click it into place.

As I noted in chapter 14, Dr. Milton Erickson started a hypnosis discussion group in my living room in the late 1950s. At first, I loved hosting that group; after years of feeling out of place in Ohio, I was pleased to be at the center of the action in Arizona. But as I neared the end of my pregnancy with my fifth child, I needed rest, and the boisterous discussions about the nature of consciousness going into the late hours every Tuesday were starting to get to me. I was no longer participating in the conversations, and I just wanted to sleep. One night I told Bill and Milton, "That's it. The discussion group needs to find a new home." I was pregnant and tired, so I wasn't particularly nice about it.

They grumbled a bit—I think that Bill, too, liked playing a central role in the important discussions that were happening, and Milton wanted things to continue as they always had—but shortly thereafter, they found a more formal location in which to host the group. The move prompted a greater discussion about the group's long-term intentions. That led key members to form the American Society of

Clinical Hypnosis (ASCH). To this day, the ASCH is the largest organization for health and mental health care professionals working with hypnosis in a clinical setting.

The boundary I set was part of my soul's journey; in that moment, I needed to mother the baby growing inside me and prepare my body for birth more than I needed to listen to long debates about the unconscious mind. But it was also a part of Milton's soul's journey, as well as those of the other souls who were affected by the work of the ASCH in the decades that followed. My decision created a temporary crisis around where they were going to host the meetings, but it was the best thing for the group overall. That's how strong boundaries work: they contribute to the good of the whole.

Setting boundaries isn't always easy. I didn't like being the complaining pregnant wife in that situation, just as Bill and Milton didn't like being kicked out of their comfortable meeting space. In my better moments, I've been able to use a little humor to soften the blow.

Things reached their apex back in Ohio when I found I could hardly go grocery shopping without being approached with a medical complaint. One Saturday morning I was at the local supermarket with all four kids in tow—Bill was away, I was exhausted and at my edge, and the children were extra wiggly. A patient saw me in the cracker aisle and made a beeline for my cart. I sighed, thinking *here we go again.*

Shockingly, Yvonne didn't bring an easy, surface-level complaint to me—she began telling me about a gynecological infection that had been going on for some time, including all the details at full volume. It was the 1950s, and although I have no problem discussing gynecology with patients in the clinic, the cracker aisle seemed an odd place to do it. My older boys roughhoused on the floor, but my younger two sat in the cart, listening to all the details and blinking their wide-open eyes.

When she got to the details of her bodily fluids, I could see that my oldest son had started to listen. I'd had it. "Well, Yvonne, why don't you just lie right on down," I said, gesturing toward the supermarket floor. "Drop your drawers, and I'll be happy to examine you right here." I smiled sweetly at my patient, ready to make good on my promise, and reached into my purse as if looking for my tools. The two boys froze in midwrestle—they knew that tone of voice, and they always had their ears pricked for a scandalous word like "drawers."

Yvonne turned bright red. "Here?" she asked, looking around.

"Or you could make an appointment for Monday," I offered, as if it were an equally good idea.

"Oh!" she cried. "Oh yes, I think I'll do that."

"I'll see you on Monday, then!" I called as I pushed my cart toward the produce, my shocked two eldest following behind snickering as the younger two giggled in the cart. I like to think that the humor softened the boundary I set—and at the very least, it marked an occasion my first four children would never forget.

I suppose part of the reason people warmed up to me so much in that town was that I gave my patients what they needed. I couldn't always solve their problems, but I became a steady presence in their lives. I went from being outright rejected to being so present that I had to start setting boundaries just to survive.

What we offer to community is as important as what we get from it. It's easy to forget this; many of us tend to think first about what's in it for us. But we gain a lot from offering up what we have and sharing. So how can we get started? How can we offer the best of ourselves, contributing to the collective life force in any situation?

Chapter 23

THE POWER OF LISTENING

Connecting with Margaret was one of the things that got me through those long, busy years in Ohio. She lived in Pittsburgh, just two hours away, which was a blessing. She, too, was raising small children and working full-time in health care. She'd trained as a nurse at Johns Hopkins and, like all us Taylor kids who had gone into medicine, was interested in furthering our parents' views of health and well-being. We had plenty of things in common to bind us together.

We saw each other as often as we could and set our kids to play; then we'd get to talking. I'd bring my high energy and renegade ideas to the conversation, and she'd bring her quiet sensibility and pure sweetness. My older sister was just the kindest, most loving friend I ever had. Sometimes I'd get all fired up about something and she'd just bat the eyelashes of her big blue eyes at me, letting me calm down on my own while she listened. Between meetings we'd often connect by phone. I'd give her a ring, and she'd hear me out; then she'd tell me what was happening in her own life while I returned the favor.

I spent a good deal of time listening to my patients in turn. I really took the time to hear what they had to say, not just about their physical ailments but about what they were struggling with in their lives. Many of them, especially the women, had never really been heard by someone whom they perceived to be an authority figure. They struggled at first to speak their truth, but as they grew comfortable with me, things started to shift.

The skill of listening has served me my whole life, because it's often the best way to start interacting positively with community. Truly listening helps us understand one another's perspectives and struggles. Our listening to others makes them feel less alone—and the act of listening makes us feel less alone. It's one of the most important things each of us can do for those around us.

My older brother Carl understood this well. After a robust childhood spent teaching me how to throw a punch and teasing me for being a *dhamar dhol* ("clumsy bucket" in Hindustani—a slight aimed at my gangly arms and legs), he went on to attend Harvard Medical School. He practiced medicine in Panama and India before returning to the United States to found the academic discipline of international health through his groundbreaking work at Johns Hopkins. One of his many projects, Future Generations, worked with local communities to improve health outcomes for women giving birth in rural provinces in Afghanistan. We were both in our eighties when he called me up and asked if I'd like to help.

"The trouble is, *Dhamar*, these women won't talk to anyone without their husbands' permission, and even then they're fairly quiet. We need to get in there and understand how they're giving birth so we can see what's going wrong. The infant-maternal death rate is shocking in some of these communities, and I'm sure there's more than just sanitation issues and poverty at play. But you're a good listener, so maybe they'll talk to you."

I agreed, and shortly thereafter, I found myself on a flight to Afghanistan. Since childbirth was attended largely by women, my colleague Dr. Shukria and I targeted a number of villages, inviting two women from each one to attend a residential program. Getting women to sign up for the program wasn't easy—in fact, when we asked to speak with women, many men didn't want to send their wives. When we recommended that they send their mothers-in-law instead, the men were happy to comply.

For a week, we all lived in a house together, getting to know one another. My colleague and I asked the women to tell us their birth stories, to see if we could identify what was going wrong. It was profoundly powerful just to listen to those women, many of whom had never had a chance to speak about the challenges associated with pregnancy and childbirth and whose stories had never been heard, even by other women in their community. In doing so, we showed them that they were important and that each of their stories was important, too.

Once the women started talking, it was easy to understand what was going on; some of them were even able to figure it out on their own. The practice of fasting during labor was weakening the women, making it harder and sometimes impossible for them to push on their own during birth. Unsterile cord cutting exposed the infants to infection. Those were simple practice shifts that could easily be implemented to reduce the death rate. Since we had listened to them, they were willing to listen to us.

Dr. Shukria and I provided them with simple information about sanitation, nutrition, anatomy, and the like. Then we sent them back to their villages to spread the information throughout the community. When women know something, they teach one another. Within weeks, the information we gave them spread throughout the rural areas by way of the existing community network. All that was needed was for each woman to speak and the rest to hear her.

Kind souls such as Carl, Dr. Shukria, and the millions of international aid workers bringing health care to the far reaches of the globe show us that the most important thing we can often bring to others is our presence. Our first role in Afghanistan was to listen, not to fix. I firmly believe that giving those women a safe space in which to talk about their experiences at the beginning of the process was as important as the education and resources we gave them later. We had to trust that our listening was important.

In return, the women had to trust that what they had to say was important, too. Most of them had never discussed their birthing process. Many had never openly talked about the children and pregnancies they had lost along the way, the friends they had seen die in childbirth or shortly thereafter, or the medical conditions such as untreated perineal tears and fistulas that many of them bore as mothers. They hadn't realized that the information they had would be valuable for us or for one another.

Yet in many other ways, the women I met in Afghanistan were perfectly clear about community. I noticed that they leaned on one another a lot. They worked together, cooked together, shared things, and asked one another for what they needed. They welcomed me into their community, even though we didn't share language, culture, education level, or economic comfort. Instead, we leaned on the connections we had: motherhood, birth, and our roles as grandmothers raising the next generation. We showed up with what we had, found connection, and created a new community together.

I was particularly struck by the power of what we had built at the week's end, when some of the women invited me on a day trip up into the mountains. It was a long journey by donkey, and though I'm still pretty tough, at eighty-six I was worried about how my body would handle bouncing along the trail. One of the women saw that I was struggling to stay upright and wanted to help. She reached up and grabbed me by the only harness I was wearing at the time: my bra. There I went, up the mountain, with a bunch of Afghani women, a donkey, and a hand firmly secured around my bra strap.

In community, this is how we support one another—however we can. When we show up for each other with what we have, we get juiced. When we receive connection openly, without fear, there's no mountain we can't climb—donkeys, bra straps, and all.

Aligning our life force with community in this way has a profound effect. It opens us up to possibilities we may never have considered. Life itself rises up to support us through community. When we most need it, it sends helpers, or human angels, our way.

Chapter 24

ANGELS APPEAR

Deaconess Hospital is a pioneering institution: founded in 1888, it was the first general hospital in Cincinnati, Ohio. But when I went to start an internship there nearly sixty years later, it had not yet employed a female physician. I had always known I would have to create my own path as a woman in medicine, just as my mother had done before me. Yet since most of my experience came from my all-women's medical school, and since women were being welcomed into certain areas of the workforce during wartime, I hoped that I would be welcomed into my role as the first woman doctor at Deaconess.

That hope was dashed to the ground almost immediately. There was no place for me to stay when I was on call, so although male doctors were given a room to sleep in, I had to bring in a pillow and blanket and sleep on an X-ray table. I was excited about the internship because it included several months in obstetrics. But then, for several more months, my internship was in orthopedic surgery. That was when I ran into real trouble, because the head resident of the surgery department, who would serve as my boss for those months, seemed to have already decided he didn't like me.

It was one of the first times, but not the last, I encountered explicit gender discrimination as a woman in medicine. The head surgery resident made it clear that he didn't think women should be doctors—especially not pregnant ones. I had been married to Bill for a few months when I started my internship, and we were eager to start having the six kids we had planned. When my first pregnancy began to show, the head resident made his opinion known. He started scheduling me for surgery at 7:30 in the morning, which meant I'd have nothing to eat beforehand because the cafeteria didn't open until 8:00. Then I noticed he was giving me the longest and most difficult orthopedic surgical procedures. My morning sickness became more intense, and I worked as hard as I could to hide from him how ill I felt. In return, he seemed to be working to make my life more difficult, paging me over the intercom for every small issue or task that arose, ensuring that I could rarely get time to rest my head or even my feet.

Seeing that, a few of the nurses supported me. So did a kindly woman named Lucille whose job it was to clean the floor at night. She was so kind that she even covered for me once when I hid in a closet, getting sick in a steel tray meant to hold surgical tools. The head resident paged me just as I finished, and I panicked, not knowing how I could clean up after myself in time to respond. As I opened the closet door, there was Lucille. She insisted that I let her clean up while I went to attend to my supervisor's newest whim.

I hung in there, toughing it out the best I could. As he became increasingly aggressive about his dislike, I continued to strengthen my resolve: not only would I finish the internship, but I would do so while showing them all that women—even *pregnant* women—were just as capable as men of practicing medicine.

Then suddenly the schedule, posted each week on a chalkboard on the surgery floor, started mysteriously changing in my favor. My name appeared next to shorter surgeries scheduled at more reasonable times of day.

The head resident confronted me in a hallway one day, furious. "Why are you changing the schedule?" he demanded.

"I'm not!" I said. It was true—I had no idea who was changing the chalkboard. It felt as though the universe was responding to my prayers. I wasn't surprised, but I was grateful. Someone cared and was looking out for me, even if I didn't know who it was.

Many people have experienced this same feeling. In the years after my parents moved to India, my father's younger sister, Belle Taylor, who was inspired by my mother, went to osteopathic medical school herself. Since Aunt Belle was unmarried, she was what we called at the time an "old maid." Despite that, and despite the fact that it was the 1920s, she came to India to start her own missionary work. Eventually she quit the mission and ended up a few hours away from my parents, where she ran an independent orphanage she started herself.

I took a trip to visit my parents in 1969 and went to see Aunt Belle at the orphanage. Many of the children were working on a big project, making clay bricks and setting them out to dry in the sun. I asked her what the bricks were for, and she explained that they were for a new cowshed. The orphanage was constantly low on food to feed its many hungry mouths, and Aunt Belle had decided that a good milk cow could be the answer to their problem.

"But you don't have a cow," I said slowly, looking around to be sure I wasn't mistaken.

"Not yet, we don't," Aunt Belle said. "But that's how faith works. Bet your buttons, if we build a cowshed the Lord will see fit to send these children a cow."

Over the course of several weeks, the children made enough bricks and constructed the shed. As the mortar dried in the sunlight, there was still no cow. So they created a feeding trough, filled it with hay, and waited.

A few days later, a cow came wandering into the yard, her udders heavy with milk. She smelled the hay and walked right into the shed! Aunt Belle fell to her knees to thank the Lord for sending her such a miracle. Minutes later, she was back on her feet and back to work. She was grateful that the cow had showed up, but she wasn't the least bit surprised.

When we develop a give-and-take relationship with the world around us, we begin to find support nearly everywhere we look. We put good energy out, and we receive it right back again. Like Aunt Belle, we can come to lean on this. Since we are the ones creating our community and the ones making it strong, we can trust that it will show up for us in our time of need. This requires faith—but not necessarily of the spiritual or religious sort. Whether we put our faith in something higher, as Aunt Belle did every day of her life, or whether we simply put faith in ourselves and our ability to create a supportive social structure, the efforts we put toward creating community contribute to our collective life force. This enables the universe to rise up to support us in return.

Aunt Belle's unwavering faith that her Lord was supporting her had an enormous effect on me—as did my mother's and my father's faith. I was raised by adults who gave to their community and expected the same in return. That turned me into a person who looks at the world this way: as something of which I am an integral part and that I can therefore trust completely.

When Bill and I were in medical school, we didn't have two pennies to rub together. Yet I wanted us to host Thanksgiving in our new married home, so I invited some friends from the hospital.

On Thanksgiving Day, we all went to a football game. Afterward, we were planning to take our friends back to our place for the holiday meal. I confessed to my friend Alice at halftime: I hadn't cooked a thing! We didn't have enough money to make an extra grocery run, so I told Bill I'd just send a prayer up and hope for the best. He shook his head, but he trusted me: when I had a hunch things would work out, I was often right. As a last resort, I was planning to serve peanut butter sandwiches.

As I finished explaining, Alice looked at me in horror. "Peanut butter sandwiches?" she asked. But I just smiled because I didn't think it would come to that. Somehow, I believed in my bones that something would come through.

We were still hoping for a miracle when we got back to the house. As I opened the door to the dining room, I saw a full Thanksgiving dinner set out on the table: stuffing, mashed potatoes, gravy, and a roast turkey in the center. The table had been beautifully set with my own finest settings. Alice looked over and laughed. "I knew you were pulling my leg, Gladys!" she said.

"I wasn't!" I said. "I don't know where this came from! I mean it!"

Just then, I saw a note on the counter. It was from the neighbors upstairs. They had been cooking dinner and been about to eat it when they had received word of a family emergency, so they had all rushed to the airport. They hadn't wanted the food to go to waste, so they had brought it down to us.

Though the family emergency that pulled them to the airport was a coincidence, the fact that they chose to donate their meal to us wasn't. We knew the neighbors and were friendly with them. They could see that we were struggling newlyweds without much family in the area, and I suppose they liked us. Faith was what allowed me to sit at that football game without a care in the world: not just faith that the universe would take care of me but faith that I had created the right conditions for it to do so. The truth is, I would have been proud to have served peanut butter sandwiches: it was what we had, and it would have been enough. But by connecting with the power of community on all levels, I made space for a miracle to occur—and it did.

If you feel unsupported by those around you, it may be worth it to ask yourself: Are you truly supporting them? Are you contributing to the collective life force or pulling from it? Are you able to maintain strong boundaries regarding where you put your attention and still find the friend in everyone? Are you offering joy and positivity to the world around you? Can the community trust in you?

If the answer to any one of these questions is "no," how can you expect the collective life force to support you back?

Community is a give-and-take relationship. Through our individual connections, we create our own network of support—one that works on all levels. I've seen time and again that when we commit to our own life force and feed it through community, angels appear to ease us along the path. It's as if life itself is rising to support us.

It turned out that it was one of those angels who was rearranging the names on the schedule at Deaconess Hospital. I didn't think too much of the changing chalkboard; all I knew was that I must have treated someone well, and they were treating me well in return. (Either that or, like Aunt Belle, I could consider it a blessing from the Lord.) Frankly, I was too tired and overworked to pay it much mind, so I just thought, *thank you*, and tried to use the extra sleep to help me better serve my patients.

Then, late one night, I was paged to go help a patient. I got up off the X-ray table, put my pillow and blanket away, and tentatively opened the door to the hallway. There I saw Lucille standing on a chair next to the chalkboard. She was carefully erasing my name from the 7:30 a.m. surgery slot and replacing it with another intern's.

I sneaked back into the X-ray room without her seeing me—it was clear that she wanted to do it in secret, as it would likely cost her job if she were caught. Quietly, I said a little prayer that someone might show her the same kindness. After a minute or two, I opened the door again and saw her pushing the cleaning cart at the far end of the hall as if nothing had happened.

From that day forward, I went even further out of my way to treat Lucille with all the kindness and respect she deserved, and I promised myself that if there was ever anyone I could help in the same way, I would do it.

When we contribute positively to our collective life force, our individual life force benefits. We find greater purpose and meaning in our days. We understand not only *that* we are part of a greater whole but *how* we are part of that whole. We align with what life intended for us to do all along.

Practice: Weaving Together the Fabric of Life

1. Think about your friends, coworkers, family, and neighbors—the people you see most often in life. Let yourself wonder: *In what ways is my community working? In what ways is it not working?* Do you feel a sense of connection? Do you rely on one another?

2. Start remembering times when you have felt truly supported by your community. This could be something simple such as being helped with a household task, being given a friendly shoulder to cry on, being given a ride to the mechanic, and so on. Let yourself remember how it felt.

3. Then allow yourself to recall times in the past when you offered your time or support to others. Think of any small action that brought someone joy. Remember how it felt to see their smile.

4. Next, ask yourself: *What relationships need my love and tending?* You can think of your love as concentric circles that radiate out from your heart. Whom can you call or connect with? Whom can you forgive? Which relationships deserve better boundaries? How can you find the friend within everyone—even someone you don't like? How can you enrich your relationships and weave the fabric of life together more tightly?

5. Now weave the fingers of your hands together in front of you, as some do in prayer, and remember that your love is your deepest prayer and truest expression of your life. Allow your hands to feel connected and supported. You can weave your fingers together like this whenever you need to remind yourself of the love of those around you.

SECRET V

Everything Is Your Teacher

Chapter 25

A LESSON IN EVERYTHING

Turning toward life is a process. It can take years, even decades, to fully make sense of ourselves and our role in the world around us. This process is made up of tiny moments—minuscule choices that we get to make over and over again. We may ask ourselves: *How am I going to handle this? And that? Where is the opportunity to accept what life has offered me and make the best of it? How can I open myself to that opportunity, even if it scares me, even if it pushes me to my absolute edge?*

We live our best lives when we approach life with curiosity and a desire to learn from everything. I believe that this is part of the point of life—to learn, to grow, to evolve in response to our experiences. Certainly, we get the most out of life when we extract lessons along the way. Life always has new teachings to offer us if we can find the courage to look for them.

Finding that courage is often our greatest challenge.

Decades ago, at the age of sixty-nine, I found myself in my backyard late one night. At the time, I was living more than an hour from Phoenix, and the stars lit the sky from horizon to horizon, highlighting the cacti in relief. Saguaros stood staunchly, their prickled arms pitched at right angles, while spindly ocotillos splayed their many limbs toward the stars above. And there I was in a robe and a pair of worn-out slippers, my arms reached upward as well, as if to demonstrate my disapproval of fate. I felt abandoned, betrayed, forgotten, like an old coat hung on a peg and left behind. I stood there in mourning, in disbelief, my head tipped back as I howled at the sky.

I'd been wearing Bill's too-big slippers all day. Though I'd always had big feet, they rattled around like pinballs in those old things, but I shuffled back and forth around our home, slapping the soles against the tile floor as I walked. I wanted to feel what it was like to walk in his shoes, literally. I wanted to understand what was happening in his soul's path to cause him to make the choices he had made, to upend my life so completely and cause me such agonizing pain.

It was without a doubt the hardest phase of my life. I'll tell you more about it soon enough. But first, I want to be sure you understand: I'm not under the illusion that this fifth secret is easy. I don't think that looking for the lessons in life, especially when we feel wronged or unlucky or just flat-out *mad*, is a simple thing to do. It's a commitment. It requires discipline. We're going to falter, fall to our knees, mess it up along the way—that's just about guaranteed.

Yet it's one of the most important things we can do in our soul's journey. When it becomes habit, it can even be joyful; the hardest moments of our life will still hurt, but looking for the lessons in them helps us process the lesser challenges more easily. When we turn toward life, we realize that it is turning toward us in return. Life is always trying to show us something. It's communicating with us through the events, people, and ideas that show up in our lives, offering us an opportunity for gratitude.

Are we listening?

Let's start with a challenging but less earth-shattering example. Just a few years ago, decades after I clomped around in Bill's slippers, I made the difficult decision to stop driving. I had always liked driving; it had symbolized independence to me ever since my very first Model A Ford that I had driven in college (it was already a clunker by then, but I loved it). Yet as I approached the centenarian mark, my eyesight began to deteriorate. I've had these eyes longer than most people have, and they simply weren't made to last forever.

I stopped driving because life communicated to me that it was time for me to do so. One day while driving a familiar path through Scottsdale, I drove over a curb. I was a careful driver, so that was unusual. I simply hadn't seen it. In that moment, I knew it was time to make a decision. Option A was to pretend that what had just happened hadn't actually happened or that it didn't matter. Option B was to hand over the keys. I thought about my great-grandchildren playing on their bikes in the road, the neighbors and friends out walking their dogs, the thousands of other drivers out there whom I didn't know but who had just as much right to be alive as I did. I handed over the keys.

Without that curb, I might not have stopped driving. It was the wake-up call I needed to make a change. Driving over the curb was a lesson from life, and I was fortunate to be able to hear and understand it.

I've been seeking out lessons from the world around me for most of my life. That's why my fifth secret for you is: *Everything is your teacher.* **When we look for the lessons, we move our attention away from our suffering and direct it back toward life.** Everything in life becomes a teacher. Seeing everything this way helps us make our life a living, breathing process. It calls us to engage and interact with everything—absolutely everything—that appears on our path.

I say that I was fortunate to understand the lesson the curb was showing me because had I not understood that lesson, a much more consequential lesson could have appeared—one that hurt me or someone else. One of my patients, Deb, had a similar experience with her health. She was going about a normal day when she suddenly lost her hearing on one side. Hours later, it still hadn't returned. She became alarmed and went to the emergency room. At first, the doctors couldn't explain it, either, so they ordered an MRI.

When she came out of the MRI machine, there was a buzz of action around her. She was having an aneurysm! She was incredibly

lucky to already be in the hospital, surrounded by emergency special-
ists. If it hadn't been for her sudden hearing loss, she might not have
survived. That allowed her to find gratitude for her sudden deafness:
it had told her that something was wrong and had likely saved her
life. Deb was grateful that life had sent her to the hospital, just as I
was grateful that I had driven over the curb.

Lately, I've heard concerns about gratitude. In some cases, the
idea of focusing on the positive can have a negative effect, an idea
that today is called *toxic positivity*. It can come off as denial. Though
the term *toxic positivity* is relatively new, the idea of it is old.

One day not too long before I put on his slippers, Bill and I were
talking in the kitchen when he became upset with me for saying that
something was "wonderful." (Perhaps that was a sign of where things
were headed.)

He looked at me and threw his hands in the air in exasperation.
"Why do you say everything is wonderful? 'This is wonderful.' 'That is
wonderful.' How can everything be wonderful all the time? It upsets
people to hear you say that. Maybe they don't think these things are
so wonderful. Maybe you're just denying the way things really are."

I was surprised by that, so it took me a moment to respond. I've
long considered optimism to be one of my best traits. "Well," I said
slowly, "because everything *is* wonderful. That's the part I see in it. I
look for what's wonderful about it, so that's the part I see."

Bill just shook his head in annoyance.

I've thought a lot about that conversation, and if I could, here's
what I would go back and say:

True optimism isn't toxic, because focusing on the positive does
not mean denying the negative. It does not mean we dissociate from
our pain, whether it's physical or emotional, or pretend that things
are okay when they aren't. Instead, it means we look for what's wonderful anyway. We allow what hurts to hurt while continuing to search
for the lesson in it and be grateful for the teaching.

Seeing the lessons allows us to access this gratitude even in the
difficult moments in life, such as losing our hearing or surrender-

ing the freedom to drive. In fact, it's often the moments when we are most challenged—by things such as pain, loss, disappointment, and heartbreak—that confront us with life's teachings more than any other.

Though looking for life lessons enables us to connect with optimism and access gratitude, it's still a challenging task. Yet even if we can't make it *easy*, is there anything we can do to make it *easier*?

We can start with resisting the urge to fight.

Chapter 26

HOW TO STOP FIGHTING

When life becomes challenging, it can be easy to feel that the whole world is working against us. For those who don't personally connect with the idea of a mystical order, it can appear that the difficult events, people, and circumstances of our lives are evidence that we're simply unlucky—or worse, for those who see life as divinely intended, as punishments that prove our unworthiness. Such challenges naturally inspire resistance in us.

Yet they continue to arise our whole life long. Though *what* challenges us and *how much* we are challenged varies greatly from person to person and from community to community, no one—absolutely no one—escapes the fact that life is hard. We just have to make a small but pivotal shift in perspective: from fighting to keep life out to welcoming it in with open arms.

As a young girl, I was a fighter. I was good at fighting, and once I repeated the first grade, I had plenty of opportunity to practice. My older brothers had taught me how to wrestle while Margaret and Gordon watched with wide eyes, and I used my new skill set to become fiercely protective of myself and my family. The other kids responded to that by bullying me for nearly everything about Taylor family life, such as our dusty seasons in the field and my parents' commitment to working with people society scorned. Even in India, we had life experiences that were far from common, and as much as I loved my childhood, every kid wants to fit in.

One day, a diplomat's daughter teased me because my mother worked alongside my father. Little Claudia Knowles stood there with her thin blond hair tied up in perfect hair ribbons and her prim British accent and insisted that there was no way my mother could be a doctor. "Surely she's a nurse. All women with *jobs* are nurses." Her voice sneered over the word *jobs*, as if she were describing a rat or a cockroach. "And most aren't even that—they're proper mothers who stay at home and host teas."

I don't remember what I said in response, but I'll never forget her look of shock as I punched her squarely in the nose.

In short order, I was scrabbling with boys on the playground, exchanging comebacks with girls after school, and catching even more pointy British noses with the solid right hook my brother Carl taught me. One girl, her hair in perfect ringlets, got it after mocking the clothes I insisted upon choosing myself, much to my mother's chagrin. Others called me stupid and sang mean songs to help their rejection sink in.

Then one morning I woke up and realized that besides my siblings, I didn't have a single friend. It was sometime shortly before puberty, around the time most kids become conscious of their social standing, and I suddenly recognized the tragedy of my situation. I lay there in bed and admitted to myself that if I didn't make a change, I would be friendless for my whole life. "I've got to stop fighting," I thought to myself. "But how?" I was as opinionated then as I am now, and I didn't want to be a pushover.

I started thinking about the people in my life and wondering which one of them fought the least. Maybe I could figure out how they managed to find a different perspective.

The answer came to me quickly: my mother. She *never* fought other people. She certainly didn't scrabble in the dust; she didn't even argue her disagreement verbally. And she was no pushover! She was able to accomplish what she wanted to in life, but she did it without fighting.

I thought about the way she managed to approach every situation with delight and humor. Even when she disagreed with something someone had said, she continued to be curious about the person and consider that perhaps he or she had something else of value to offer. She was wise in the particular way that people with deep self-love are: strong, yet flexible at the same time, like the bolts of soft silk I saw on our family trips to the market.

I realized that if I wanted to enjoy my life and the people in it, I'd have to quit fighting the kids who teased me and interact with them more positively instead. I'd have to act more like my mother. I'd have to bring humor, wisdom, self-worth, and every other tool I could find to the people who challenged me so I could meet their animosity without fighting back.

That moment was pivotal for me. Since then, I've built strong connections with others, and most people find it hard to believe that there was ever a time when I struggled to have friends. Looking back more than ninety years later, I realize that it was a change in perspective that affected me in many ways. It wasn't just other kids I learned to stop fighting; it was *life itself.*

Lying there in bed, I began to redirect my energy toward engaging with life instead of battling it, especially when things got tough. From that moment forward, I began to let life teach me, even when I disagreed and even when it hurt. I started directing my energy toward finding what each challenge had to offer me, instead of draining myself by struggling to change what was happening. In doing so, I became strong, yet soft and flexible. Like silk. Like my mother.

There's so much in life that we don't understand when it's happening. In bed that day, I thought I was just resolving my social challenge; I knew it was an important shift in thinking, but I had no idea how important it would become. That simple concept—*stop fighting*—would go on to become one of the greatest understandings of my life. It came from pain. It came from loneliness, rejection, and fear that things would always be as they were. Leading up to that moment, I didn't feel joyful or light; I felt heavy and dark. Yet that was the moment when everything changed for me.

This is the truth about so many things in life: it's challenges that push us forward. I think about Dr. Milton Erickson, the great psychiatrist and psychotherapist, whose little meetings in my living room morphed into a proud consortium of professionals working with therapeutic hypnotism. Milton's interest in consciousness—the conscious and unconscious mind and how they work together—began in the long months he spent in bed fighting polio as a teenager. He experimented with his theories on himself, using the muscle memory stored in his unconscious to teach his paralyzed and atrophied legs to walk again. In the decade before I met him, he struggled with post-polio syndrome and had to test his theories again to remain on his feet. At the time, those couldn't have been easy experiences; he surely suffered. Yet the lessons about the mind and the nervous system that he gained through his solitary inquiry helped him unlock his greatness. They led him toward a professional field he loved, where he created a legacy that lives on to this day.

Milton learned to turn toward the virus living in his nervous system and ask what it had to show him about the power of the mind. I had to learn how to turn toward my friendlessness and ask what it could teach me, which in the end was to stop fighting my life. Our experiences were very different, but our shift in perspective was the same: we both had to redirect our resistance and focus not on what we'd lost but on what we had to gain.

Without challenges, we aren't truly alive. I'm concerned to see how many parents today try to protect their children from challenges. When we don't let kids take risks and see things that scare them, we damage them. We cut them off from the real world. This hurts them because it keeps them perpetually children, and it hurts parents because it forces them to keep playing the role of protector forever. That doesn't mean we should expose them to everything;

the polio vaccine was a very good thing for the world, and even my mother forced us kids to wear shoes to protect us from scorpions and snakes. But a little bit of danger is good for kids.

Numerous spiritual paths refer to the connection between growth and suffering. We can't stop ourselves from suffering—and we shouldn't stop our children all the time, either. Children need to know that they can grow and heal, and they have to hurt just a little bit for that to happen. As adults, we need this, too; we need to demonstrate through our own growth how to redirect our energy back toward life after a period of pain.

Redirecting energy like this is a choice that requires us to bring our very highest selves forward—especially when things are hard. Doing so has an immense effect on how we experience life: it helps us reengage with the world around us, give the best of ourselves, and receive the best in return.

Making that choice sometimes requires great effort by our conscious mind. So what should we do when we're so challenged by life that we lack the juice to put forth that effort? That's when we can allow the other parts of our consciousness to lend a hand.

Chapter 27

THE ROLE OF DREAMS

When we ally with our conscious mind, it becomes a wonderful collaborator. Positive thinking has the power to make dramatic changes in both our lives and our health. Yet try as we might, we can't always overpower our resistance to challenge right away. It takes time to make doing so a habit, and even when it is a habit, the sudden events and repeated circumstances that bring us to our lowest points can make it more difficult to deal with our minds.

This is why the moments when we face our biggest challenges are some of the most important times for us to investigate our dreams. Think of it this way: even if you can't do anything about your conscious thoughts, you can still go to sleep and see what happens.

Dreams are important throughout life. They are the way that our subconscious, and often even our unconscious, speaks to us. Sometimes powerful beings such as guides, ancestors, and others we may have known in past lives appear in dreams. Other times, dreams can show us the answers to our problems or at least help us see them in a new light. Whether you are a person who believes that dreams come from somewhere or someone other than yourself doesn't matter much. Regardless of whether they signify help from beyond or simply help from the obscure recesses of ourselves that are generally harder to access, they can be of enormous assistance.

People have been using dreams for guidance for thousands of years. Joseph, son of Jacob, was famously guided by dreams in the Old Testament (or the Torah). Dreams help shamans from many different cultures, and dream interpretation is a foundational part of both Freudian and Jungian branches of psychology. Many people have had dreams about future events, including President Abraham Lincoln, who is said to have dreamed of his own assassination in the nights before it took place. Using dreams as a source of wisdom goes across cultures, across religions, and across time.

I have always used dreams to guide my choices and decisions in life. I encourage my patients to do the same. This doesn't mean we should always interpret our dreams literally. Dreams often use symbolism to make their point. If you're not a person who is drawn toward symbolism in waking life, it can make you feel vulnerable to try to interpret dreams' symbols on your own. You may wonder "What do I know about interpreting dreams?" The key point to understand is that since a dream came from *your* mind (or your guidance, your highest being, your ancestors and past lives—whatever fits your system of belief), *you* are the one who is best suited to interpret it. Your dreams are made precisely for you, which means that the symbols you find in them are very likely to convey their intended meaning to you. If you think your dream means something, it probably does.

One woman came to some workshops on holistic health I gave sometime in the 1970s. Her story was heartbreaking: she had caught her husband abusing one of their two boys. She had immediately divorced him, and he'd gone to prison for the abuse, but later, he had been released without her knowledge and had kidnapped their sons. By the time we met, it had been several years that she hadn't seen her boys. She had no idea where they were. At that point in time, there were very few ways to track down people who had run off like that, so she had more or less resigned herself to the idea that she would never see her children again.

Hers was a truly impossible circumstance. I wasn't about to tell her to forgive her husband or get "through" her grief or try to heal or any of the rest of it. Some things are just terrible, and there's no way around it.

Yet I could help her get through her days. One of the most concerning symptoms of her grief was that it was impossible for her to sleep, as she kept having a repeating nightmare. Night after night, she encountered her ex-husband in their kitchen standing over their boys. In the dream, she would pick up a butcher knife to stab him. But at the last moment, he would always hold up one of their sons, and she would end up stabbing the child instead. This nightmare tormented her for years.

As we worked with the pain of what had happened to her and her sons, she saw that the dream was trying to show her what directing her energy toward her ex-husband was doing: it was creating a repeated cycle of hatred, and what her sons needed was her love. She came to the realization that her hatred for her ex-husband was consuming her. It took up an enormous amount of her energy—energy that would be better spent sending love to her children, who were likely facing impossible tragedy as well. Her hate couldn't help them; only her love could.

I'm not suggesting that I found her a solution; I didn't. If I could have changed anything else about the situation and brought those boys home, I would surely have done so. Yet I did the one thing I had power to do: I gave it some context in her soul's journey. I helped her extract a lesson in love from what was otherwise pure pain. She had to really search for the lesson, but when she did, she saw it and it lifted her up. That was part of how she managed to move her focus back toward the love she felt for her sons. It didn't change how she felt about the situation, but it changed where she put her life force, which was precisely what her dreams were asking her to do. It directed her energy back toward something constructive.

Many of my patients have received such guidance from dreams. People receive guidance about their purpose, their health, their decisions. Dreams bring clarity to questions that feel too big for the conscious mind to handle.

So what's the best way to go about receiving guidance from your dreams?

Start by asking. Request a dream, and be ready to receive it. Remember, this doesn't need to be something spiritual or supernatural, if that doesn't work for you—it can be merely psychological, as you ask your sleeping self to show you what you don't yet understand.

Once you've received a dream, look for symbols. What do they mean to you? Did anyone visit you in your dream? If so, what does that person represent for you? Oftentimes, it's the tone of the dream that has the most to show us—the actual contents of the dream may make no sense at all, but the underlying feeling that accompanies them can answer our questions and help us find the perspective we seek.

Over time, that perspective will change. That's a good thing! Recording our dreams can help us make sense of them later, and the more often we record them, the more likely we are to remember them; just the act of recording dreams sends a signal to the subconscious that they are worth remembering. Whether through journaling, visual art, or voice recording, try taking note of important dreams that come your way. Doing so will help you extract more meaning from the messages you receive.

It's good to do this throughout our lives. As I grow older, I find that my dreaming becomes richer. But it's especially good to do this when we come up against issues that affect us repeatedly. Whether they're physical, emotional, or spiritual issues—or, more often than not, all three—we all come up against chronic challenges of some type.

Chapter 28

WHEN YOU JUST KEEP HURTING

When we choose to see everything as a teacher, we learn to trust the process, even when our current circumstances feel impossible. Doing so is a worthy endeavor. If we're lucky, we slowly learn to shift our perspective automatically, without having to think about it. This is a particularly useful skill when we face a challenge that repeats itself.

There's a science to how this works. Studies have found a correlation between repeated negative thought patterns and management of chronic pain.[18] This is why cognitive behavioral therapy (CBT) is now so often recommended for people with ongoing disorders such as rheumatoid arthritis and migraines, both of which are severe, episodic, and often debilitating forms of chronic pain. These chronic conditions include repetitive symptoms that often follow the same pattern each time. Yet changing how we think about pain can interrupt that pattern ever so slightly, and that has an important effect.

Some people with chronic pain are even able to let their pain inform a certain activity that gives them meaning. My eternally positive friend Evelyn, who walked the Camino de Santiago trail, as I explained in chapter 18, has lived with chronic pain for years. She has learned to paint her way through flare-ups, swirling colors with her brush when it feels like too much. She keeps painting until she feels what she thinks of as the "ting"—the joy, the bliss, the release— and then she puts her paints away and goes on with her life. She calls these works of art "pain-tings." Evelyn's outlook demonstrates what's possible when we open ourselves to a shift in understanding. I believe that's one of the main lessons that chronic pain has to teach us: the power of our own perspective.

Another patient, whom I still coach today, is experiencing macular degeneration. Her slow loss of eyesight is something that most people would find terrifying. Yet in the absence of physical sight, she reports that she's able to perceive more. She once said to me, "I may be los- ing my sight, but I'm not losing my vision." She's learned to embrace the process, attuning to the input her other senses can provide. She's become clearer about what she wants to accomplish with the eyesight she has left. This doesn't make losing her sight any less tragic, but it does provide a useful context that connects her challenge to her purpose. Not only that, it inspires others. My century-old eyes stopped working well enough to allow me to drive, and now they're making it increasingly difficult for me to read. This gives me a reason to think of her statement about vision a lot. While staying at home, I listen to audiobooks and imagine what I'm going to do and create next. I have more time to envision my next steps, and I'm grateful for that.

Sometimes repeated challenges arise to show us what we have been neglecting or the parts of ourselves we weren't able to nurture in the past. I recently worked with a patient, Sarit, who came to see me in my home.

Sarit had a creative career for which she was well suited, yet it required her to spend long hours at the computer. She had ongoing pain and tension in her right shoulder that was making it increas- ingly difficult to work, especially as her online time increased during the Covid pandemic. She sat in the chair next to mine, surrounded by the relics of my life, and asked what she could do.

I had questions for her in response. I asked her whether she had ever used her right shoulder frequently as a child or teenager, and she explained that she had spent many years pitching softballs as a kid, always with her right arm. Her face tightened as she said that, so I asked to hear more about her memories of softball. Had she liked her teammates? Had she liked playing?

She looked over my shoulder at a plant on the windowsill, as if she were trying to remember. At first, she was quick to stress that she had liked the game, but then she softened. "I guess it was really more of my dad's thing than mine. He wanted me to play, and I wanted to please him. I got better and better at it, it's true—but I don't know if I would have *chosen* that particular sport in the first place."

I found that statement odd. "What would you have chosen, then?" I asked.

Sarit's face lit up, but then her cheeks fell slightly. "Oh, surely I would have been a dancer. I always dreamed of it," she said. She went on to explain. There was a well-known dance studio by her school, one that many of her friends had attended. But Sarit's parents had worried that the studio encouraged concerning messages about body type—things they didn't want their young daughter to internalize. By keeping her out of the dance school and pushing her toward softball instead, they unintentionally led Sarit to internalize a different message. "I guess I thought that since they wanted me to play softball, I wasn't good enough to dance. That probably wasn't the message they meant to send, and as a parent, I realize that now. But it was the message I got at the time." She looked back at me as she said that and pressed her lips together hard.

I suggested that Sarit add dance to her regular repertoire—not dancing to perform but dancing for no reason. She started integrating five-minute dance breaks into her workdays at home, and slowly her shoulder began to release. Her false identity—as a softball player who "wasn't good enough" to dance—was what had been causing her pain. In fact, her pain was trying to show her that she *could* dance. As an adult, Sarit was now completely in charge of her days. The only one stopping her from dancing in adulthood was herself.

That day in my home, Sarit learned that she could choose to get up and dance whenever she felt the tension in her shoulder increasing. The tension was an invitation, and she chose to accept it. Chronic issues work precisely like that; they give us the chance to practice finding and making choices repeatedly.

Many patients with chronic illnesses have come into my office over the years. These illnesses, which are hard to measure and often even harder to treat, are the ones most often seen in the general medical community as warranting holistic treatment, because it's clear to everyone that they involve a complex set of factors that are individual to each patient. (I tend to believe that nearly all illnesses function this way, but not everyone agrees with me on that.)

I love working with patients who have chronic symptoms because, in many cases, it's easiest for them to make the connection between their symptoms and their life. After approaching numerous "quick fixes" that didn't work, they're ready to consider things from a broader perspective.

For several years, I found myself working regularly with two middle-aged women who both had chronic symptoms of lupus. Treating their cases side by side allowed me to view their symptoms and approaches to resolving them in tandem, noticing that what helped for one didn't necessarily produce the same effect in the other.

One of those patients, Janet, seemed to be making some headway. Over time, I watched her grow in the way she dealt with her symptoms. Lupus pushed her to try different diets, adopt new sleeping and exercise routines, and adjust her social life to a gentler rhythm. She was learning from her lupus how to live a more balanced life. She often came into my office so bright and cheery that it was almost surprising when she listed her symptoms—terrible headaches, joint pain, inflammation—because I just couldn't imagine that she faced such difficulties in her daily life and still managed to maintain such a positive attitude.

The other client, Laura, felt stuck. I don't just mean that she herself felt stuck; I also sensed a stagnant energy around her, as though there were something she couldn't or wouldn't release. It isn't my intention to be dismissive of everything she was going through; lupus is a very challenging condition that deeply affects the lives of those who have it. Yet Laura seemed to somehow be turned toward her lupus more than she was toward her life. Accordingly, though everything I tried with Janet I also tried with Laura, Laura's symptoms never seemed to abate.

As I worked with both of them, I found myself desperately wishing that Laura could adopt some of Janet's attitude. Both women were in pain; both women were deeply challenged by the inflammatory pattern in their bodies. Yet Laura seemed to be suffering, while most of the time, Janet wasn't. Janet's lupus seemed to integrate with her life force instead of draining it. She was learning life lessons from her body, such as how to find purpose and flow, to say "*Kutch par wa nay*" to the foods and activities that weren't serving her, to practice loving self-care, and to lean on her community. She was allowing it to teach her how to live her best life.

I wondered how I could teach Laura what Janet seemed to comprehend.

To understand how these two women were approaching their experiences so differently, let's look at what we go through when shocked by pain. There are times when we are blindsided by what life throws our way. We receive a scary diagnosis, life takes a difficult financial turn, or a relationship suddenly falls apart. How can we find the teaching in our moments of greatest pain? How can we convince ourselves to look for the lessons available to us when our hearts, bodies, and hopes feel irreparably broken?

Chapter 29

IN THE IMPOSSIBLE MOMENTS

It's time for me to tell you about my most impossible moment. I was nearly seventy years old when I received the greatest test of my fifth secret that I've experienced thus far.

Sometime when I was in my early eighties, a person I met while traveling said that since I was so happy, I must have "had it easy." I laughed as I answered, "Honey, if you only knew!" I had just emerged from the hardest decade of my life. Not only that, my pain had been extremely public. It seemed that everyone in my community knew about the ins and outs of what had happened: how Bill left our partnership—both our marriage and our business—to be with a nurse from our clinic.

What everybody didn't know was that it wasn't the first time he had considered ending our marriage, because I had told hardly anyone. There had been another nurse back in Ohio, though he had never confessed it, and though I'd had my suspicions, I'd believed that what he told me was true. All I knew for certain was that he suddenly announced that he'd been carrying divorce papers in his briefcase for six months and he wanted me to sign them as soon as I could. At the time, we'd had four children under ten, and divorce was far less common. I'd been shocked—I hadn't done anything wrong. I'd spent the long years while he was in the service raising the kids and running our clinic without him while he was stationed out of state. It had been particularly hard because our nurse had a sick mother, also out of state, whom she regularly traveled to visit—a story line I was suddenly beginning to question. I'd explained my side of things: that we'd committed to each other that day at the altar. We'd followed that commitment for twelve years thus far; we'd made our life together, had had our children together, and I wanted to stay together. Whatever was wrong, we would fix it.

We traveled all the way to Kansas for a week of intensive marriage counseling, and I tried, as the therapist advised, to be more docile or some other word I didn't understand. I got the message that I was too headstrong for Bill. My ambition was coming off as domineering. The way Bill and I had always interacted—sharing ideas, having long philosophical discussions, working alongside each other as business partners as well as spouses—was unhealthy, because it wasn't the way husbands and especially wives should behave with each other. It was the 1950s, and I had internalized a lot of ideas about women and submission. I'd thought when I'd married Bill that he was a different sort of man who wanted a different sort of wife, but it appeared I'd been wrong about that. It was a disappointing and confusing realization, but I took it to heart. I stepped back a bit and let him lead the way.

Shortly thereafter, he led us to Arizona and to the beginnings of our interest in alternative healing modalities. *Aha!* I thought. *So he does want a partner, not just a wife!* Our working relationship became stronger, as did our friendship. Both grew immensely during the decades that followed. Together, we led workshop after conference after symposium, photocopying newsletters to send around the world and stamping each envelope by hand. The clinic we ran was well known and successful, and we had many friends in the community who looked to our marriage as a pillar of what was possible when two great minds unite. Our one-on-one talks went late into the night, and in them, we pushed each other to new understandings and novel possibilities. We were a great coparenting team and joyfully brought two more children into the world in Arizona. It seemed to me that the marriage therapist's advice had pushed us toward the next step in our marvelous life together; as long as I let him win most arguments and take the leading role in our public life, my boisterous and curious nature was welcome. Our children grew up and got married, and we became grandparents. Life went on.

Then one day, thirty-five years after his original petition for divorce, Bill began to push for a nurse at our busy clinic to become the administrator. That would require me to step down from my leadership role. The idea seemed strange—though she was a good nurse, she wasn't a natural leader by any means; in fact, hardly anyone liked her. The only one who seemed to like her was Bill. They'd go on professional trips together and sometimes work late at the office. I'd asked him several times about his friendship with her, which had grown considerably over the years she'd worked with us, but he had always laughed off my concerns.

I balked at his proposed administrative shift and suggested he go up into Oak Creek Canyon, our favorite spot for soul-searching, to consider whether it would be her or me—at the office, that is.

All that weekend I prayed that the good Bill McGarey I knew would come to his senses. I had a good many conversations between Gladys, the small part of me who still wants to fight, and Dr. Gladys, the wise counselor who sets her straight. Gladys was afraid, but Dr. Gladys was certain that she would get through whatever happened next.

What happened next was just about the worst thing possible, or so it seemed at the time. Bill came home and abruptly handed me a letter—one he'd already handed to all six of our adult kids, as well as the board of directors at our clinic. It explained that his soul needed to be alone and that as a result, he and I were divorcing. It was the first I'd heard about it, but by then, everybody else knew. It was the right thing for him to do, Bill explained, an integral part of his soul's path. My soul's path wasn't considered, I suppose. We had been married for forty-six years.

He moved into the guest room that night, and shortly thereafter, he moved out.

He took just about everything he owned with him when he went, perhaps trying to prove that he wasn't coming back. One of the few items he left behind was his old pair of slippers. As I wandered around the house in the days after he left, moaning and sobbing, trying to keep my body moving so I didn't lock up in fear, I kept eyeing those slippers. It felt as if they were winking at me.

Finally, Dr. Gladys piped up. "Now, Gladee, Mama always said to understand a person, you've got to walk in his shoes. Put Bill's shoes on. Try to understand."

It took just about all the life force I had to follow her advice.

I walked in those slippers all day and long into the night, pacing around the house, wandering aimlessly out into the yard. And that was where I ended up, howling.

Several months after that, Bill sent me another letter. It came in the mail. It was an invitation to his wedding to that same nurse turned administrator—the one he had put in charge of the clinic that had once been ours, the clinic I'd been forced to leave so they could run it together. It turned out that his soul didn't need to be alone all that long.

I had always been willing to believe his story that they were just good friends, despite my suspicions. And I felt we'd had a strong marriage anyway, one in which we had truly been partners in all aspects. His choice to leave had destroyed it, and sending that invitation made the reason for his choice plain. The decades we'd been married felt like a farce. I had never felt so hurt or humiliated.

He sent the invitation to my new clinic, of all places. I gritted my teeth and got through the day. But on the long drive home, my hands gripping the steering wheel as I barreled down the highway, I started to scream. It wasn't the agonized lament that had been pulled from me in the yard; it was something even deeper that started as a groan, moved into a growl, and grew into a roar. It was rage, pure and simple—the same rage that I'd put into my right hook on the playground, the same rage that had demanded I fight to survive. I screamed at God, I screamed at Bill, I screamed at the universe, I screamed at life itself. I screamed for almost ten minutes straight. I felt I couldn't stop. I realized I didn't want to.

And then, just as suddenly as I'd started screaming, I stopped.

In that moment, I realized that some unknown thing was coming for me. Dr. Gladys showed up and took control. Up until then, as far as I had been concerned, my future was being married to Bill, but now a future I had never imagined was opening in front of my eyes. And in that future, there was something worthy of my gratitude. I had an opportunity up ahead. The experience had something to teach me—even if I had no idea what that "something" was yet.

I remembered my mother, soft and strong like silk. I remembered what the other girls had called me in college: "Happy Bottom," a euphemism for a less polite play on my name, "Glad-ass." I couldn't change Bill's decision, but I could change my response to it and be glad anyway. "There's something to be grateful for, even here," Dr. Gladys counseled, and Gladys steered the car back onto the highway. A few days later I put in a request for a new license plate, one that stayed on the back of my car for years to come. It said: "BE GLAD."

There I drove, crisscrossing the greater Phoenix area with the public dissolution of my marriage in full view, being grateful despite it. I'd park my car in the lot of the brand-new clinic I'd started with my daughter Helene, the one we'd managed to get a private loan for despite my being over the common age of retirement. I listened to the part of me that knew what to do, found the teachings, and discovered that life went on.

No matter how shattered we may be, no matter how much we may feel that we don't know how to handle what's happening, there *is* some part of us that knows exactly what to do. There's always some small voice that can guide us through managing what life throws our way. I call my wiser self Dr. Gladys. You can call yours whatever you want, but I promise that you have one. Each of us has the wisdom to get us through the impossible moments. We must believe that.

When we face our absolute hardest challenges in life, it's an event like mine in the car, one in which we choose to seek out wisdom and look for the teachings no matter how much it hurts, that reignites our life force again. We feel it when it happens. There's a lift, a hop, a sudden sense of freedom in our movement. It feels immensely powerful because it is.

And then life continues, just as it did before our impossible moment. New challenges crop up, and we continue to shake in our resolve to choose the light. Healing doesn't happen all at once in the moment of choice; it's an ongoing process. But as we move forward, something magical takes place: We begin to extract more and more from the pain of the past. We realize that we can keep gaining lessons out of our old hurts, and they can affect how we approach what comes next.

Chapter 30

LESSON AFTER LESSON

Seeing life as a teacher means that as long as we're alive, there are more lessons to gain. There's no rush; the lessons come in their own time.

Shortly after Bill left, my daughter-in-law Bobbie, who is a minister, told me, "This is part of the tapestry of your life. If you look at it too closely, you'll only see the individual threads and knots—that's the back side of the tapestry. But as you move on, you'll begin to see the whole picture."

She was right.

It took many years for me to fully extract the lessons from my divorce. Though my attitude toward finding the teachings changed in a moment, I didn't actually receive them all in my car that day—not by a long shot.

In the years that followed, I came to see that Bill's wanting to be with someone else was reason enough for us not to be together, even if I wanted to stay married to him. I understood that the years of pushing myself down to be the demure wife I thought he needed had helped at first. In fact, that may have been part of the greater reason for the first shake in our marriage: it had caused me to step back, which had allowed him to lead us both toward the next step in our lives and careers. If he hadn't have been dominant, would I have been open to all of the people and ideas he brought into our home? If he hadn't pushed to move way out west, would I have agreed to go?

But over time, putting my needs second to his had taken a toll on my soul's mission. That, coupled with old beliefs I still held on to about not being smart, had caused me to keep him in the lead role in our work together, long past the time when it was useful. I'd let him write the newsletters, I'd asked him to rewrite my speeches, and I'd been the "and Gladys" in "Drs. Bill and Gladys McGarey."

My soul had immense amounts to learn from being Dr. Gladys on my own. And though my divorce felt like the end of my life, I am here to tell you thirty-four wonderful years later that it wasn't. In fact, my life got a whole lot better from there. I started writing books, leading in my own right, and I became who I had always been meant to be. I ran the new clinic with my daughter Helene for another quarter century.

In that time, I faced numerous other challenges. The greatest by far was the death of our headstrong and brilliant daughter Analea, my beloved Annie Lou, who died of cancer in her fifties. All four of my siblings passed on in their time, as well. Losing people is one of the greatest tragedies we experience. Death itself is a challenge, whether it's the massive loss of someone very close to us, the death of a pet, or even the small sadness we experience when we find a dead bird beneath a glass windowpane. But we must learn to give the death of others space in our lives while still finding gratitude, because we will all have to experience it sooner or later. Death is part of daily life; it's there as life ebbs and flows. We have to experience the grief of death, or we cut ourselves off from life. We have to let our children experience it, we have to turn toward it our whole life long, or we close ourself off from the realities of being alive.

My divorce was its own kind of death, and the lessons I gained from it guided me through the periods of grief that followed it. "BE

GLAD" remained with me—not just on my license plate but as my philosophy for life. That moment in the car didn't change everything, but it was certainly the start of a greater shift. It took the same lesson I'd learned in childhood and deepened it, showing me the extent of what is possible when we choose not to fight.

Yet it still took me a good decade to work through every last bit of anger and betrayal. I eventually came to realize that I still loved my husband—in fact, I still do. I still love the Bill McGarey I married. He was my partner and friend. His soul and my soul were meant to walk together, and we completed that walk.

As I processed it further, I began to receive new lessons. For years, I'd identified as Bill's wife. In the early years after he left, I still held on to that identification—I was Bill's first wife, Bill's divorced wife, the one he had left. Working through that new identity took its own time. Once I'd gotten through it, I could embrace the role that had always been available to me: Bill's friend. That's what I consider us to be today, even though he passed away years ago. We're friends. We're two people whose lives were intertwined and who will undoubtedly meet again in some other format in the lifetimes to come. We learned so much together. We surely aren't done yet.

Often in life, it's outdated identifications that cause us pain. Seeing life as a teacher is important here, too, because it frames each of us as a student. This is perhaps one of our most important identifications in life. We may be a daughter or son, a father or mother, a sibling or friend; we may be religious, spiritual, or atheist; we may come from this or that country or have a political identity that is important to us. Yet understanding ourselves as a student of life is the most important identification of all. It gives context to both our struggles and our joys.

In fact, it allows at least some of our struggles to *become* our joys.

I learned this lesson once again from Janet and Laura, the two patients with lupus whom you met in chapter 28. It turned out that the two of them had very different ways of identifying with their lupus. One day, I had a treatment session with Janet just a few hours after a

challenging session with Laura, whose symptoms had remained un-
changed. Thinking of Laura and witnessing Janet's success, I asked
Janet if she identified with her pain in any way.

"Oh, no," she answered. "I have pain, and I have lupus, but pain
and lupus are not me." She described how she dealt with a flare-up
by putting her "friend" in a chair across the room. She was a teacher,
and she always kept an empty chair in the classroom. Whenever her
pain spiked, she'd look at the chair. "You sit there, pain, and don't
you dare get up," she'd think to herself, "I'll just be here." There they
would sit—in the room together but separate.

I found Janet's particular approach so remarkable that the next
time I saw Laura, I asked her whether she identified with her pain.
Laura was quick to respond that she was proud to be living with lupus;
she had overcome a lot. "In fact," she said, gesturing out the window,
"I even got a vanity license plate like you did, Dr. Gladys. See?" I
looked out into the clinic parking lot and there was her car, parked
just a few spaces away from my own. Laura's plate said "LUPUS."

I sat there, stunned. She had missed the point of my license plate
entirely: I had identified myself with what I wanted to emulate, while
she had identified herself with what she was struggling to overcome. I
didn't want to suggest that she was to blame for the pain she felt from
lupus. Yet I suddenly understood why her suffering was so severe.

Kindly, I tried to lead her toward separating her identity from her
symptoms. I wanted her to understand that though she *experienced*
lupus, it was important for her not to *become* lupus. I wish I could say
that she improved in response to that session, but in fact, she didn't.
As long as she was my patient, she continued to suffer greatly from
her lupus and continued driving around in the car that reminded
her of that fact.

If you find yourself dealing with something that seems impossible
or screaming at the universe as I did after Bill left, it's important to
acknowledge the intensity of your challenge. First let yourself feel
its strength. Then allow the intensity to help you recognize that the
moment is potent. You're being presented with an important oppor-

tunity, and it's a good time to start asking some questions. *What do I have to learn? What does this experience have to teach me? How else could I view this?* Then, if you can, BE GLAD! It's okay if you can't feel grateful for the situation yet; be grateful for your decision to try. Test out a smile, and if it's possible, push yourself to laugh out loud. Shake your belly. Use your voice. Do it even if nothing is funny and you have no idea how on earth it's all going to work out. Remind yourself that this doesn't mean you are to blame; it means that you are the only one who can possibly flip it around.

It may also help to ask yourself, as Janet did, *What else is in the room?* Look around you—is it just your pain, your anger, your grief, or is there something else there? Is there a chair for your challenge to sit in? Is there any other furniture, or are there any other characters, such as joy or curiosity or wonder? What else is in the room with you—and where are you in all of it? Are you only this terrible thing that has happened, or are you somehow something more?

Activating such a shift in perspective takes practice. It's awkward the first few times and may even feel forced. But the more you do it, the more automatic it will become. Eventually, this simple concept has the power to change your life, providing you a much more pleasant and purposeful experience of being alive.

When we see that everything is a choice and each moment is an opportunity to learn, we stop holding back. We understand that life is meant to be lived, through good times and bad, right up until the very last moment.

Practice: Finding the Teaching

This exercise isn't always easy. It's something we practice over and over again in the hope that we may someday succeed in it. Be gentle and kind with yourself, always.

1. To ease our way in, we'll start with a more comfortable memory. Think back to an event that taught you a lot in your life. It could have been an easy lesson or a moderate one, but don't choose a hard lesson here; choose something that doesn't activate a strong emotional reaction.

2. Then let your mind run through the lessons you learned from that event and the positive things that came from it. Really feel its positivity; let it pour over you like sunlight. You're gathering strength for the next part of the exercise, so allow yourself to bathe in the positivity first.

3. When you're ready, allow your mind to wander to something that is hard in your life right now. It may be related to physical health, emotions, relationships, finances, the world around you, or anything else. Pick something tough—something that feels unfair or undeserved.

4. Next, begin to consider this difficult thing from all angles. Start asking yourself questions such as *What could this mean for my soul on a larger scale? What could I be learning here? What wisdom could I get from this extremely challenging experience? How could it shift my relationship with the past, the future, or my life today? What could it be here to teach me?* Imagine yourself years from now looking back on this challenge—what you might have learned from it and even how it may have helped you grow and change, leading to a richer life. Though at times it's hard to push through pain or distress, try, as there are gifts in the pain.

5. Then ask for a dream to help show you what you aren't seeing. Go to sleep, let your subconscious inform the process, and proceed to step 6 once your dream has arrived. Record your dream as soon as you wake up so you get all the details—even the ones that don't make sense.

6. Consider what you recorded about your dream. How might you interpret it? How might the different characters, locations, phrases, actions and/or events from the dream help you understand your challenge?

7. Whatever answers you find, send them gratitude. It doesn't mean that you are grateful for what is happening. It means that the fact that you can find even one small part of it that is positive is a miracle. No matter how insignificant it may seem, be grateful for any lesson you find, and be grateful to yourself for being brave enough to seek it out.

8. After you are finished, place your hands together, palms touching, thumbs against your heart. This version of prayerful hands or, as some call it, "*namaste* hands," is a universal symbol of gratitude. In Hindustani, *namaste* literally means "I bow to you." In this exercise, we are bowing to life as our teacher.

SECRET VI

Spend Your Energy Wildly

Chapter 31

ENERGY AS INVESTMENT

Since the moment in my childhood when I learned not to fight, I have spent each day of my life directing my energy toward what feels blissful and good. It's turned into a long life and a remarkably happy one—happy enough, at least, that many people have asked me what I'm doing differently from others. My answer is hard to put into words. It's taken me over a hundred years to explain it.

The reason it's hard to put into words is that at the heart of it, the answer is about energy.

Life itself is energy.

I've passed through many years, treated many patients, and stood on many stages trying to explain this without making it sound too "out there." The truth is that it's not that out there; it's right here. The first law of thermodynamics states that energy is not created or destroyed, it merely changes shape. The world that we know is energy. It's all around us; it's in us. Just as a mushroom, a flower, a caterpillar, or an elephant is made of energy, so are we. Our life force is the directional aspect of that energy; it's how that energy moves through us. It's where it comes from and where it's going.

Living well, therefore, is merely a game of learning how to steer our energy toward life. It requires us to direct our loving attention toward the pulse that ebbs and flows within us, finding the precise rhythm of how that energy moves and immersing ourselves in it. When we do so, life comes alive. It becomes a joyful interaction. We find our bliss day by day, moment by moment, in the flow of love. I'm living proof.

To do this, we have to rethink everything we've been taught about what life is. Life is that which reaches for more life. We're therefore called to embrace the wild rhythm in our souls and seek out the reason we are here in each moment, finding what juices us again and again—and offering our life force to that.

Throughout these pages, you may have noticed that I refer to life force, energy, and love somewhat interchangeably. That's because for me, they're all pretty much the same thing. My first secret taught you to find the life force within you; my second secret explored why it's so important to find where that life force is flowing. My third secret explained that life force is activated by love, because to a degree, it *is* love. My fourth secret helped you see how we amplify love and life force through community. And my fifth secret urged you to remember this in even the toughest of times, so you can gain lessons from them to help you move forward.

My sixth and final secret is: *Spend your energy wildly.* When we fully integrate the first five secrets, we are able to consciously invest our life force in that which gives it back to us, tapping into a continuous flow of positivity and light. To put it plainly, **when we align our energy with life, we create a give-and-take, sharing relationship with the source.** We no longer have to try to make our own energy, which is a losing battle anyway, because energy is not created or destroyed. Instead, we invest the energy we have in life. Then, when we're running low on what we need, we simply borrow it back.

The reason I have saved this secret for last is that it's the trickiest to explain. It isn't something we understand as much as it is something we *feel.* It requires us to tap into our deepest knowing, the kind that bypasses the thinking mind and goes straight into our bodies and souls. I've carefully named this secret "Spend your energy wildly" instead of "Spend your energy wisely," because although wisdom is a beautiful thing to follow, far too many people associate this old adage with an overly cognitive type of wisdom. This secret isn't about that type of wisdom; it's about the wisdom of our wildness, the wisdom of our bodies, the wisdom of the cycles of the universe. By focusing on turning toward that which increases our energy, we naturally turn away from that which drains our energy without giving it too much of our attention.

We live in an era in which our individualism is celebrated. Modern culture promotes self-importance and independence. We may wonder, *Who am I to be connected to something greater and more important than myself? Does that mean I'm not great or that I'm not important?* This way of thinking encourages us to hoard our resources. We're told to conserve what we have, to dole it out neatly so we can be sure we'll have enough.

Yet looking at the world this way creates a tightness and a holding in that resist the flow of life itself. I promise you that if you're reading this right now, your heart is beating, your blood is flowing, your breath is continuing to move in and out, and that means you still have energy left to spend. When we get locked up in fear and stop using the energy we have, we block not only the life force moving out from ourselves and into the world but the life force that's meant to come back to us.

Our fear of not having enough goes back generations. Recent studies on epigenetics, or the way genes turn "on" and "off" in response to lived experience and are then passed down in that state, show us that we are still responding to the challenges our ancestors faced, even if they aren't our own challenges today.[19]

Many of our ancestors really didn't have enough. Our parents and elders may have passed their anxiety onto us in childhood. Their fear thus became our fear.

This fear is at the heart of the question many patients ask me: they want to know how I managed to get so old, because they're worried about running out of time. This is the same worry that many people have about food, attention, and money: *What if there isn't enough?* Yet living from this fear simply gives it more strength.

If we really want to tap into our life force, our goal must be to flip things back around. We need to ask ourselves: *What do I have enough of? What can I spare? What can I give in order to receive?* These questions can feel counterintuitive. They may even sound plain exhausting to try to answer. But when we look at our energy as an investment, something new becomes possible. Instead of seeing an empty account and wondering what happened, we can ask ourselves: *Well, what did I put into my account lately?*

Many of us have heard of the idea that when we give love away, we get more in return. Some of us even said it to our children or grand-children when they were small. Yet like most things that are designed for children, it's easy to forget that the same principle applies to us as adults. And because life force, love, and energy are basically inter-changeable, it works for all three.

It works, that is, when we start to understand *where* and *how* to spend our energy.

Chapter 32

WHAT'S WORTH YOUR ENERGY?

To get beyond the fear that we're going to run out of energy, it helps to look to where our love flows freely, without fear.

That means we have to look toward the things we love the most in the world—the things that feel good and help us grow. Then we can let that love show us the energy available to us.

Just a few months ago, I was offered access to an archive of my mother's letters to the church leaders from my parents' time in India. The letters comprised almost fifty years of monthly reports, explaining whom my parents had treated and why, detailing exactly where the money had gone, and respectfully asking for more. In 1916, after pushing for a couple of years, my parents succeeded in opening a women's hospital in what is now Uttarakhand province. It was the first in the area; until then, women could receive medical care only in the field camps because the local hospitals weren't open to them. My parents ran the hospital for nearly four years before receiving a letter from the mission saying that since the economy was suffering, there just wasn't enough money to do everything that was needed. They would have to choose: either cease their fieldwork or close the women's hospital.

The next part is a story I remember from my childhood. My mother once told me that she and my father had gone up into the mountains, walking toward the snowcapped peaks with only a mule to carry supplies and a young boy to tend to the mule, leaving the children with our nanny, Ayah, and another missionary for a whole month. When she told me the story, I assumed that I had been left behind with the others. But based on the dates of those letters, I now realize that the excursion took place during the early part of her pregnancy with me.

My parents would have known my mother was pregnant by then—they were doctors, after all, and she had carried three pregnancies already. They also certainly knew the dangers associated with the high Himalayas. They were undoubtedly tired; she was likely feeling ill, as women often do in early pregnancy; and there were plenty of things to fear, regarding both the potential loss of the hospital and the elements they would face. Yet off they went, carrying me along with them, quietly retreating to nature to grapple with one of the hardest decisions they would ever have to make.

My parents loved adventure. They loved the unknown. They loved the Himalayas. That was the love they put their energy toward as they made their decision. Surely, for many people it would be an inopportune time for a Himalayan trek—for most people from their background, *any time* would have been an inopportune time for a Himalayan trek! But for my parents, it was the best way to find the strength they needed to decide. A month after they left, they came back down from the mountains with their decision: they would continue their fieldwork and close the hospital.

My parents lived wild, incredible lives. They never stopped. They didn't conserve their energy. To the contrary, they spent every bit they had on what they loved—and nothing else.

My mother cared little for the things that were important to the other women from her culture; she tended to her clothes and appearance and was always presentable, but she held her typewriter ribbon in far greater regard than she did any hair ribbon. She continued to value humor until the day she died. Just before she made her transition, she had a bad fall. We rushed her to the hospital, and as she lay there on the gurney, writhing in pain, she still wanted to make a joke and lift our spirits. "The old gray mare just ain't what she used to be," she said, smiling up at me and my father. She did that because she understood something important: as long as she still had energy left, it was up to her to keep spending it on what brought her joy. Seeing the two of us as we looked down at her and laughed was worth it.

Spending our energy on what we love is important. It helps us turn toward life and receive the energy that is waiting for us. But that doesn't mean we should spend all our energy, all the time. Each of us has to find the rhythm that works for us and adapt to it as it shifts and changes.

Life's flow is based on rhythm. Forests have a rhythm: they burn to the ground and regrow. Bodies have a rhythm: they're born, they learn a series of lessons, and then every single one of them dies. Agriculture has a rhythm: we till the soil, plant seeds, tend, harvest, and let the ground rest. Old scriptures often reference the spiritual nature of embracing these natural rhythms, such as the idea of a seventh day of rest that is woven into Genesis. No one can decide your rhythm but you. Like my mother, trekking through her pregnancy, and like me, living big at 103, you have your own rhythm.

Rest is a natural part of the rhythm of life. The phases when our bodies are growing the most—infancy and adolescence—are when we need to sleep the most. Many plants grow the most at night.[20]

Resting is often an important part of healing, too. And I have counseled many women who are giving birth to rest and relax between contractions. Doing so makes the contractions more effective and gives the women the energy they need to continue with labor. Seen this way, it's easy to understand how rest gives us our juice.

This is true even when our rest changes over time, which it naturally does. Many of us sleep less as we age. We're often told to call this "having trouble sleeping," but I'd rather ask people if they consider it "trouble" before labeling it as such. Some people really struggle with insomnia, and there are many modalities of medicine equipped to deal with that particular issue. But others are just following their natural rhythms, and in this case, it isn't necessarily a problem.

Personally, I don't see my diminishing sleep as trouble at all! I often find myself awake at night. Instead of succumbing to anxiety about not sleeping, I use the time productively to focus on what brings me joy and happiness. I work though the things that challenge me, consider my goals and plans, and allow myself to wander down memory lane, remembering all the lovely people and moments from my past. It isn't sleeping time lost; if I needed to be asleep, my body would be asleep. Instead, it's a type of rest that rejuvenates my juice and helps me dedicate my best energy to the day ahead.

And when I do sleep, I have spectacular dreams. They have become much more beautiful and more intense as I age; I travel to new worlds and gain new insights, right there in my bed. Even when I'm asleep, I'm active. My whole body is humming with life. That's just the natural way my body wants to rest.

True rest is an *action*. It's meant to be something we *do*; it's not just the absence of doing anything at all. While resting, we're meant to think kind, gentle, regenerative thoughts about our body. We're meant to nourish ourselves, enjoying a slower pace and being fully present to what is.

This is a far cry from laziness. As I see it, being lazy is when we withhold our life force from the collective; it's when we hold back, refusing to give, refusing to participate. This drains our juice. The purpose of resting is just the opposite. When we rest, we're consciously dedicating our energy toward what's most important to us. We're reminding ourselves of our orientation: toward that which is positive and good and will help us bring our best to others. True rest honors our body and our soul's greater mission within our incarnation. Rejuvenating ourselves in this way enables us to give life our "all."

Giving it our "all" can bring up even more fear, because many of us worry that we won't have enough. Yet it's precisely in such moments that wondrous things can happen. Just as angels appear when we need them most, it's sometimes in the moments when we feel we're about to run out of something completely that it comes back to us.

Chapter 33

MAKING SPACE FOR MIRACLES

In the late 1930s, Aunt Belle hitchhiked home from India. She criss-crossed her way through the Middle East, Asia, and Europe, eventually finding her way onto a boat and arriving on the East Coast of the United States. My father's other sister, my staunch and proper Aunt Mary, drove to New York to pick her up; I guess she'd had enough of Belle's shenanigans and simply wanted to see her home. By the time Aunt Belle arrived on the dock, carrying a small bundle of clothes after having given the rest away, she was so disheveled that Aunt Mary barely recognized her.

Aunt Mary took Aunt Belle home, cleaned her up, and bought her clothes to fit a lady of her station. But throughout that visit, Aunt Belle refused to conform—just as she always had. Poor, exasperated Aunt Mary was at her wits' end. She was trying to help Aunt Belle raise money for her orphanage, but Aunt Belle just couldn't manage to impress the members of high society the way Aunt Mary had hoped she would. Sure, she could lead group prayers, talk about her faith, and explain the important work the people at the orphanage were doing for orphans, but she didn't behave the way Aunt Mary's friends were accustomed to seeing a "proper lady" behave.

One day, Aunt Belle went out for some hours and came home wearing a beat-up pair of old shoes on top of her new stockings. "Belle, what have you done?" Aunt Mary asked, throwing her hands into the air. "I just bought you new shoes! What on earth happened?"

Aunt Belle smiled and laughed it off. "Oh, these shoes will do me just fine. I made a new friend, and she needed them. She was living on the street and having a hard time. Plus, our feet were about the same size."

"Belle! You traded her your shoes? But these are full of holes. You can't possibly make it through the winter in them. However are you going to get new ones?" Minutes later, Aunt Mary marched Aunt Belle out the door to buy her new shoes once again, just as Aunt Belle had suspected she would.

In our family, everyone laughed as they retold that story—including Aunt Mary. It's an integral part of our family lore. We saw it as but one more example of how Aunt Belle lived her life: with unfailing faith that whatever she gave away with an open heart would come back to her. That was part of what we all loved about Aunt Belle: she inspired us to remember the magic that is available to us when we understand how our own energy flows with the rest of the world's. Sometimes we have to get down to the bare bones to get something in return—and it's only when we do this, really giving all we've got, that life starts to send energy back to us. It's as if the greater "bank" of the universe is asking "Do you really need this loan?" When we answer "Yes," our wish is granted.

This doesn't relieve us of our own responsibility in the matter. Aunt Belle would have lived just fine with her holey shoes, and she was willing to do so. This is what it means to take a measured risk. But certain risks are necessary to a well-lived life. If we aren't willing to risk our energy, we start to guard it. We disconnect from our own wildness. In the end, no matter how careful we are, we end up risking and losing everything to fear.

So how can we know which risks are worth taking? When is it

worth spending our energy in the hope that it's an investment that will bring us more in return?

The answers to these questions are often individual, because they have everything to do with the precise blueprint of each person's soul. We never know what tragedies or miracles will befall us. Each of us experiences incredible events in our lives, every one of them part of our soul's journey. That's why I've guided you throughout this book to understand who you are and what you came here to do, so you can contact the physician within and answer many of your own questions.

At the same time, I do have a bit of advice on the matter. There are certain things that are almost never worth anyone's energy. I hope that by this point, I've made it clear that lamenting the past, digging into self-pity, and feeding negativity are rarely useful—and then only when they help us change our present and future. My other five secrets can help you discern this, as well.

On the other hand, things that give you juice are always worth your energy. My brother Carl loved his work in international health. He continued to lecture well into his nineties, when he lived with a painful tumor. His final lecture was four days before his death in 2010.

Understanding where your life is moving and where it is blocked is essential to knowing where to spend your energy. If something feels stagnant, put your energy toward what is moving. Don't waste your energy on what's stuck.

Love is always worth your energy. Always. Lean into what you love, whom you love, how you love. Love is an endless font of life force, and it's always there for you.

Good community is worth your energy, too. My sister, Margaret, was quite disappointed when she realized that she would be spending the final years of her life in a retirement community. But then she decided to make the most of it. She made dear friends, joined the band, and drummed as Ayah had taught her to as a child. She found happiness in her new circumstances because she welcomed the community that came with it, and in the end, she lay on her deathbed singing, claiming that Ayah was at her side.

Looking for the lessons in everything guides our energy, as well. In eighty years of practicing medicine, what I have seen is that the patients who understand this the best are the patients who suffer the least. My friend and patient Bobbie Woolf (not to be confused with my daughter-in-law, also named Bobbie) is one example.

Decades before I met her, when she was just a toddler, Bobbie fell into a bucket of hot tar and was rushed to the hospital. Emergency room doctors were able to save little Bobbie's life, but she lost one of her kidneys and more than half of the other. She spent most of her early childhood in a hospital hooked to a dialysis machine with one quarter of one kidney. She was eventually able to spend weekends at home and then full days at school, but she had to wear a special device that left her with tubes dripping into maxi pads. It was difficult for her to make friends both because of her condition and because of the lack of exposure she'd had to other children. Time and again, she received the message from the medical community that she couldn't expect to live a full life.

Luckily, she didn't believe it.

Bobbie became an athlete in high school. By then her body had compensated for the empty space on one side by curving her spine to meet it, giving her scoliosis. She pursued numerous sports anyway. Her connection with the other girls on her various teams enabled her to break through the social stigma of her condition and teach them what she herself believed: that her difference was not something to be mocked but proof that her life was miraculous.

Her early struggles turned her into a remarkably self-assured person. She learned early on what is worth her energy and what isn't. She pays little attention to what other people think of her or what the medical community says about her. Instead, she devotes her life force to exploring what is possible in the body she has. She puts her love toward the friends she has made and the son she raised.

Susan, who rebuilt her spine in chapter 18, also stopped paying attention to what most others thought; their ideas hadn't helped her heal, but her own had. That gave her a deep trust in her own intuition. Late in life, long after she had retired from her teaching position, she dedicated her life force toward changing the pattern of violence in schools. She continued to find juice in her days because she continued to put her love toward that which brought her meaning, and when she finally passed away, she donated her body to science so the miracle that had taken place within it could be studied.

Each of those women used her struggles to help her identify what mattered to her unique soul. Both spent their energy wildly on that. In return, they were gifted with rich and incredible lives.

Understanding what is worth each person's energy varies from individual to individual and from moment to moment. Learning to listen to our own inner knowing is the key to discerning, in any given moment, how and where to invest our life force. And it takes truly *living* to understand this. We're meant to interact with our lives. The work of life is simple: we must try and fail until we succeed.

The truth is that I can't tell you exactly what's worth your energy—but your life can.

When we live life this way, every moment becomes an opportunity to answer important questions: *How much life force should I give to this? And how much life force should I give to that?* We find ourselves increasingly able to say "*Kutch par wa nay*" to the things that don't matter, just as my mother taught my siblings and me to do so many years ago. The process itself becomes beautiful. It brings us alive.

As we practice this, it's inevitable that we come across thoughts and things that we realize are draining our life force. In some cases, they are easy to address; we simply let those elements fade from our lives and move on. But what can we do when we identify activities, places, or even people that are draining our life force but we either can't or don't want to eliminate them from our lives? How can we find a way to shift our relationship with the elements we want to keep, without discarding them completely?

Chapter 34

FEEDING THE POSITIVE

A s with so many truths I've shared with you, it all comes down to perspective.

When I try to explain the concept of how we spend our energy to my patients, many of them immediately adopt the inverse interpretation and start thinking about how to *conserve* their energy. This misses the point entirely. It rests on a negative view. Many people are so accustomed to this negative view that they don't even realize they're harboring it—but I do, because I see everything, and I mean *everything*, in the positive.

What this means in our process of discernment is that when we identify that something, some place, or someone is draining our energy, we don't necessarily need to cut them out of our lives. Instead, we need to consciously offer them a different type of energy. We need to take the reins and decide how we are going to shift that interaction from a negative one to a positive one.

Getting through my divorce was probably the hardest thing I ever did. Long after I decided to BE GLAD, I struggled to put positive energy toward what had happened. Sure, I could put positive energy toward the rest of my life, and I could be grateful for all that I didn't yet understand, but to feel good about the divorce itself was much more difficult.

During that time, Bill and his new wife were largely not a part of my life in the physical sense. We rarely saw each other. Yet emotionally and mentally, they were very much a part of my life. I realized early on that thinking about Bill's new wife was a drain on my energy and that I didn't owe her anything anyway. I released her, *kutch par wa nay*, like flowers to the water. I don't wish her ill, but I don't spend a drop of energy on her, either. That decision alone freed up a good deal of my life force for other things.

But I didn't want to cut Bill out of my life. On the day of our wedding I had promised to love him forever, and that promise didn't end with our marriage.

I had forgiven Bill's decision. Yet I could see that my life force was still going toward him in a negative way, and I could see that I was less vibrant and alive because of it.

The Bill who had left me was with me when I went to the clinic each morning. He was with me as I sat to watch the sunset most evenings, the orange and pink glow silhouetting the saguaro cacti across the desert. The sad thing was that it wasn't even a Bill I knew. I had managed to make peace with the universe and find gladness for everything I had to learn—but I hadn't let the hurt go. My energy was being drained by the idea of the divorce, and no matter how much I tried to fill myself with juice, it was sapped back out of me again. I was devastated to think that that was what I would remember from our marriage: the way it had ended and the heartbreak that had come with that.

Then I got yet another lesson from Bill and our divorce. On the evening of my seventy-ninth birthday, I had a dream.

In the dream, all the family was gathered around the large oak table in the home we'd lived in for most of our parenting years. All our kids were there, as was Bill. My mother was there, too. She came up to me, kissed me on the cheek, and said, "Tell him he must go now."

I turned to Bill and said, "You have to leave."

He got up, kissed me goodbye, and walked toward the door. That was when I realized he was holding a hundred silver ropes. The ropes were tied around me. I found myself pulled to my feet and following him against my will. I struggled but could not get free.

Then the whole family rose to their feet as well, and I saw that each of them was holding scissors.

One by one, members of our family cut the silver ropes until I was free of them. Bill paid it little mind, as if he didn't know about the ropes, and continued walking out the door and down the driveway. He got into his car and drove away.

When I woke, I understood that the ropes symbolized negativity. They didn't symbolize our *connection*.

In the years that followed, I sent the Bill who had married me pure love. I gave him the life force that I wanted to give him. I offered love toward the memories of our marriage, the good times we'd had together, the funny things our kids had said, the triumphs and surprises in our shared career. At the same time, I stopped giving my life force toward the Bill who had left me, because that was a man I hardly knew. I put energy toward what had worked and refused to give energy to what hadn't. I consciously spent energy on Bill—but I spent the positive energy that would feed my own life force, not the negative energy that would drain it.

Today, when I think of Bill McGarey, that love is what I remember best.

This is what I suggest you do as you discern the subtle shifts in how you spend your energy. If there's a part of a certain activity that you don't like but you want to keep the activity in your life overall, adjust the energy you're giving to that part. If there's a part of a person you don't like but you want that person to remain in your life, change the way you relate to that person—both in your interactions and in your own mind and heart. Find what you *do* like. Give it your best. Offer it everything. Invest your life force there.

There are many ways to do this. One dear friend, after years of being blessed with a large yard, found herself living in a small apartment. At first, being in the apartment bothered her. She missed having a garden to tend. She missed looking out her window toward the neighbor's yard and was bothered that her new view was a sea of bricks and concrete. So she bought one houseplant, then another and another. She built a small planter on the balcony and planted cherry tomatoes. She gave her tiny container garden everything she had, filled her view with green, and came to love her new home just as she had the other one.

A patient of mine, Eric, found himself reevaluating his career after the Covid pandemic. He'd liked working from home, it turned out, and didn't want to go back to the office. But his manager felt differently, and when the work-from-home order was lifted, Eric had to return to working in the office from nine to five. He wasn't able to leave his job from a financial perspective, so he asked himself what he'd liked most about working from home. He came to see that he'd loved the relationships he had built with his neighbors, connecting with them in small ways as they went about their days, and that he had enjoyed spending more time with his dog. He also deeply disliked the morning meeting in his office, which he found dry and devoid of meaning.

Eric explained this to his manager, and together they set up some lunch-hour social events so colleagues from different departments could connect outside work. The social connections they formed made it more meaningful when they bumped into each other around the office and inspired a much livelier morning meeting. Eric found that when he put his energy into connecting with his colleagues, the meeting was less boring; instead of just waiting for it to be over, he actually started looking forward to it. And most important, the manager agreed to let Eric's dog come to work with him a couple times a week, which brought joy and delight to everyone in the office.

These examples remind us that it often isn't what's on the outside that needs to change for us to be happy; more often than not, it's an internal shift in attention that sets us free.

Chapter 35

SHIFTING YOUR ATTENTION

When something catches your negative attention, you're faced with a choice: Will you move away from that activity, person, thought, or place, or will you stick with it? If you decide to stick with it, the only thing to do next is to find what's positive in it and feed that. Pay attention to what *does* matter. Don't sit there fighting your life with negativity—instead, give it your best.

Some years before we met, Barry had been diagnosed with chronic fatigue syndrome. He was by then in his seventies and newly a grandfather. Chronic fatigue is often caused by a latent virus, such as Epstein-Barr, or tick-borne bacteria such as those that cause Lyme disease. But plenty of people have these viruses and bacteria in their systems and *don't* suffer long term; somehow, their energy is directed differently. That's why when I treat these illnesses, I don't just look to the pathogen but also to how and where the patient is directing his or her energy.

In my office, Barry sank low into his chair. He seemed older than someone in his seventies to me—not physically, though of course most of his hair was white and his skin was looser than I supposed it had been in the past.

He described his symptoms to me. As much as he slept, his energy didn't seem to return. He found himself sitting in his living room recliner more often, watching the daytime news. Meanwhile, his wife went about doing all the things they'd used to do together on her own: tending the garden and meeting friends for their weekly bridge game. "She's a little slower than we were thirty years ago, but she's still going," he explained. "I mean, she's going in a way that I'm definitely *not* still going. She gets up in the morning and she just goes, doing this, doing that, calling her friends and chatting. And I'm just thinking, Is this it? Is this the 'golden years'? I have to wonder: Am I just old?" His eyes widened as he said it, as if he suddenly felt embarrassed to ask this question of someone twenty years his senior.

I noted how he had walked into the room: how he had dragged his feet slightly, his shoulders a bit hunched. There was definitely something going on with him. It was as if his life force was bypassing him; life was happening around him, but he wasn't a part of it, and not just because he was missing card games.

"Well, how are you spending your energy?" I asked.

Barry snorted, and his face twisted a bit. "What energy?" he asked dryly. But then he smiled and asked, "But really, what do you mean *spending* it? The doc said I was supposed to rest."

"Well, yes, but when you *aren't* resting, do you like what you do? Do you enjoy the way you spend your time? Do the things you put your energy toward return energy to you?"

"I suppose I never thought about it that way," he answered, rubbing his hands together in his lap. "I thought I was supposed to save it." He looked nervous and uncomfortable.

As I do with many patients, I started asking about his childhood. I wanted to understand the lens through which he saw life. Why was he so worried about risking his energy?

Barry told me that his mother had been very risk averse. Though today he understood that she had lived with a lot of anxiety and didn't blame her for it, his childhood had not been unlike that of my son Carl's little friend, the one who had been sent out to play in gloves. Barry's mother would shout at him to not climb too high on the play structure, and he was rarely allowed out of the house on his own—even to the front yard. He told me of one particularly strong memory of her telling him not to ride his bicycle in the cul-de-sac they lived on for fear he would be hit by a car. He had stopped cycling shortly thereafter. While the other boys had been zooming around town on their bikes, he had mostly stayed at home.

"I liked being alone, though," he explained, smiling. His expression seemed genuine. "I just didn't like feeling left behind. Looking back, I think I wanted to explore."

As a teenager, Barry had spent more time with other kids. Though he had liked that, too, he had found himself drawn to do whatever they did. One friend was on the basketball team, so he had joined the basketball team. Another friend had gone to a certain university, so Barry had attended that one, too.

"I guess it's hard for me to know what I really like, Dr. Gladys," Barry said. "I know what other people like, and I know what I'm supposed to like, but I don't know what *I* like. Plus, I don't want to disappoint anyone—especially not my wife."

Together, Barry and I decided that he would need to find out, even if it disappointed his wife.

We started discussing how he could shift his thinking about how he spent his energy, instead of trying not to spend it at all. He immediately noted that watching the news wasn't serving him, so he started to use the time in his chair to write stories from his life. Once he had written all the stories he could remember, he started inventing new ones, imagining the places he might have gone if he had explored more and what he might have done there. He enjoyed reading these stories aloud to his adult kids and his young grandchildren.

Since his schedule as a retiree allowed it, he started taking entire months off, going off by himself into a cabin in the woods or taking a solo beach vacation. He made trips to parts of the state he hadn't seen before and even booked an international tour. Eventually, Barry's wife tired of caring for their yard alone, and together they made the decision to downsize so she could tend to a smaller garden while he traveled.

About a year later, Barry came back to see me and shared that he had much more energy. During his trips on his own he had started cycling again for the first time in more than sixty years. He enjoyed working on and refining his writing. He still rested more than he had at forty, but he no longer felt fatigued. Instead, his life felt full, and he was using his downtime to prepare for the rest of it.

Furthermore, he was excited to say that his wife was much happier, too. In the years he had spent in his chair, she had taken on more and more of their joint responsibilities, and she, too, had grown bored with their routine. She was happy with their smaller house and garden. She enjoyed having time to herself. And she was relieved that *her* life force wasn't being put toward making Barry happy, because he was finally taking responsibility for that. Their marriage was undergoing a small renaissance, Barry explained, and even their kids had noticed how much more alive they both seemed.

In his seventies, Barry started spending his energy in the ways that brought him joy and meaning, and as he did so, he found that his energy began to return to him. He started to like living again, and his body felt better and better. He never did return to playing cards, though. It turned out that bridge simply wasn't fun for him. His wife brought her sister in to be her bridge partner, and Barry spent the time they played together going for long bicycle rides in the sunshine.

If you are struggling to find energy to tackle the tasks life brings you, it may help to follow Barry's example and ask yourself whether you really want to do those activities in the first place. Do they bring you joy? Do they drain your energy or amplify it? Do they increase your love, give you juice, get you involved with the people around you, and help you feel alive? If the answers to these questions don't come easily, consider my other five secrets. Allow them to help you identify the feeling of life force flowing within you. Then return to the questions and see if anything changes.

Once you've done that, it's time to start making choices: What do you want to do? How do you want to go about doing it? What do you still want to be, explore, learn, or discover?

It may also help to mix up your routine a bit. Look for the rhythm of life and follow it. You may notice that making small shifts in your days can bring you renewed support in recognizing that you are the source of your own energy and that your activities and relationships are there to assist you in increasing the life force you already have. Look for any false beliefs you may hold regarding avoiding risks or not having enough. Are they serving you? How could a shift in perspective help you adjust them?

When we do this, we get back into the flow of the natural world around us. We realize that the sun rises each morning without worrying whether it will run out of energy, because it knows it is the source, and it knows it is never ending. As long as there is life, there is energy. It's up to us to invest it in what matters.

Practice: Embracing Your Life

1. Consider the activities, people, and places you've put energy into throughout your life. What has drained your energy? Where can you invest your energy and receive a return?

2. Then try to get out of your thinking mind for a moment and *feel*. Let your thoughts wander over those same activities, people, and places in your life, but this time, instead of just thinking about them, *feel* them. Does your energy flow freely or shrink back? Do you feel an increase or a decrease in your life force? This is subtle, but practicing the other exercises in this book has prepared you to answer these questions. What does your *deepest knowing* tell you?

3. Based on what you felt in step 2, consciously pick one activity, person, or place that brings you more energy. How could you invite

more of that into your life? Could you practice that activity more often, give that person a call, or spend more time in that place? Find one small shift you could make and move toward it.

4. Thinking of step 2 again, consider the people, places, and activities that drain your energy. Look for at least one thing you can just stop doing completely, the way Barry stopped playing bridge. Pick something small to start. Your deepest knowing will guide you. What would it take to just give this up? Could you do it with gratitude and love?

5. Then consider the things that are draining your energy but that you don't want or aren't able to release. How can you change the way you spend your life force? Can you change the way you think about that person, can you adjust the way you spend time in that place, or can you shift the type of energy you put into that activity?

6. Once you've contemplated these things and perhaps even jotted down a few notes, open your arms wide and imagine yourself embracing the force of life. Feel life's boundless energy moving out from your heart and through your fingertips. Embrace your life in all of its joys and sorrows, challenges and learnings, triumphs and surprises, and be glad that you have been given the precious gift of life. You can practice this first thing in the morning or just before going to bed, allowing yourself to embrace the wildness of life all around you.

YOU ARE RIGHT ON TIME

One evening in early 1960, Bill and I attended a lecture on husband-coached childbirth. The idea was nearly revolutionary in the medical community at the time, and I was excited to sit with other doctors and practitioners on the cutting edge of empowered birth practices that put childbirth back into the hands of women, their partners, and their chosen practitioners. I was about thirty-eight weeks pregnant with my sixth child at the time. I had already been lucky enough to birth my fifth child intervention-free at home, and I intended to do the same with the baby currently residing in my womb.

I looked down at him lovingly. And that was when I realized something was wrong.

I put my hands to my belly instinctively, feeling around the swell created by his small body inside mine. My hands were trained by assisting hundreds of pregnancies, and I instantly confirmed my suspicion. My child, who in a matter of weeks would need to come out headfirst, was firmly seated on his butt. I felt his little head up around my rib cage—the exact opposite of where it needed to be.

I'd turned babies in the womb plenty of times before, but not usually so late in the process and never my own. I knew that many breech babies are born healthy. At the same time, I knew that the baby's position would inevitably complicate the labor. I wanted to get my child flipped around, and fast. As the lecturer kept talking, I worked quickly to address the situation before my concern had a chance to turn to alarm. I did what I always did when I turned a baby prenatally: I started talking to him.

"Now, listen here, little one," I communicated internally to my child. I rested one hand gently on his head and the other on his butt. "You've got to get born in a couple of weeks. It's going to be a little tough for you and a little tough for me, but I know we can do this, and in the end it's going to be wonderful. But for that to happen, you've got to turn over. We need your head down when the contractions come. We need you to turn toward life."

Simultaneously, I talked to myself. Gladys the mother was worried. But Dr. Gladys knew better. "Don't worry. There's nothing to fear here. What's happening is happening, and if it's happening now, it's right on time."

Fear tells us it's too late. It tells us that we haven't done enough, been enough, seen enough, learned enough, or made enough money. It tells us that we're behind where we should be, that others are ahead of us, or that we're running out of time. But love has its own timing. Life has its own timing. That timing deserves respect.

We see the power of time in life's most important moments. We see it in birth. We see it in death and in grief. We see it in healing.

I hope you will take the lessons I've shared with you into your life. You may relate more with one of my secrets than another. You may want to see how each one works to shift your perspective as you navigate your life. And in the process, you may come up against some common fear-based questions: *Is it too late for this? Am I too late?*

And the one that always makes me laugh these days, given my age: *Am I too old?*

The longer we live to look back on life, the more humorous the question becomes.

My bright and cheeky great-granddaughter Maggie Mae turned five a little over a year ago. She wanted a princess birthday party, with ribbons and balloons festooning the house, and she told everybody in the family what they needed to do to help her celebrate, giving each person a special task to do or role to fulfill. Her father was to clean the house, her two-year-old brother had to stay home from preschool, her grandmother was to take care of her new baby brother, and her mother was to bake and decorate the cake. After the presents had been opened, the beautiful cake devoured, and her happy, carefully orchestrated day was drawing to a close, Maggie Mae's eyes grew sad. Her family asked her what was wrong. "Now I'm five years old," she said. "All my four-year-old days are over. Now I have to grow up."

She took the growing-up business very seriously. At the breakfast table the next morning, when her father passed her the jam for her toast, she said, "I'm humbly honored by your generosity." No one had taught her the phrase or coached her to use it. It was her own adaptation to the circumstance of being five—of getting older.

I think many of us look at life and aging this way, each passing year a clarion call that announces that the fun is over, it's time to grow up and get serious. Or we reach a certain age or stage of life and feel that we've stopped growing, that healing is impossible, or that we'll never change. The funny thing about youth is that it always seems to be running away from us. Even Maggie Mae thought she was too old! We're never done growing, though. And healing is never impossible. It's always a good time to make a change.

This is why when patients come to me with a concern that they're too old, I wave their concern away. "*No one* is too old," I say. I figure that at my age, I've earned the right to say it.

As a species, we're a bit confused about age in general. We're aware that we will all eventually die, so looking at it one way, every day is a step toward that end. But over time, we start to realize that the idea that anyone is "too old" to do something is just plain absurd. It becomes laughable, like sweet Maggie Mae's serious admission that turning five meant it was time to grow up.

Can you remember the first time you became aware of your age? For most people, it was quite some time ago. Can you remember the first time you thought you were "too old" to learn to play an instrument, "too old" to go back to school, "too old" to make a career change, or "too old" to change a relationship?

Looking back, were you "too old" then?

If not, how can you be sure you're "too old" now?

In caring for pregnant women and attending their births, I encountered plenty of women who had been told they were too old to become mothers. One such woman was my colleague in medical school. After five miscarriages and in her late forties, she got pregnant and gave birth to a ten-pound baby boy. I've now seen so many examples like this that I no longer think they're miraculous. In fact, there's family lore that one of my great-aunts had a baby when she was sixty and another when she was sixty-two! I chalk this up to another one of the universe's mysteries.

This doesn't mean that every woman will give birth to babies after a certain age—or at all, for that matter. These are mysteries that are out of our hands. We can't control things like this; we can simply surrender to them with hope and gratitude, and see what comes.

Part of what makes mysterious happenings possible is our belief that we don't know everything, that there are things greater than we are that cannot be explained. I cannot overstate the importance of keeping a sense of wonder about the world as we age. It is what keeps us young. Our souls benefit from our holding on to the idea that we don't know what's going to happen next.

I wonder what would happen if we flipped our perspective on the phrase "too old"? Instead of thinking we are wasting time *not* doing whatever it is we'd like to do, what if we consider that we have in fact been working on it all along?

I like to joke that I keep telling God my schedule, but he doesn't listen. The universe doesn't understand my timing any more than I can understand the divine timing.

This is just the way time works.

I've counseled many a pregnant woman who gestures to her swollen ankles, points at her giant belly, and demands, "I want this one out! Now!" My answer is simple: "That baby will come out when it's good and ready. I promise."

The truth is that although it's sometimes necessary to bring a baby out before it's ready, it's not usually in its best interest. Important things are happening in there, even if we don't know what they are.

In today's world, we're very focused on manifesting. We're most interested in the moment when something comes into being—when we put out a book, buy a house, or receive an award.

But this is only one side of what's happening. In the deep energetic underground of the universe, the things we will eventually manifest are undergoing gestation. We're gathering experiences to put into the book. We're working to save money for the house. We're learning and doing the things that are going to inspire someone to offer us an award.

I call this process *femifesting*. It's what's happening in the womb, and it's also happening to our life force throughout our lives. We're stocking up, preparing, learning. A huge part of turning toward life is embracing femifesting, even when we don't understand it.

Sometimes we're good and ready but someone or something else or even the world itself is femifesting, preparing to receive what we have to offer.

When Aunt Belle finally left India for good, she went to a church service where she met a minister named Ed who was a recent widower. I don't think Aunt Belle was even thinking about marriage at the time—she was well past what was considered the "prime" age for getting married and had never shown much interest in men. But she and Ed fell in love, and a month later, they held a joyous wedding. Belle and Ed started a whole new chapter of their lives together.

Had they met earlier, Ed would have been married. Had Belle been younger, she might not have been interested in settling down at the edge of New York City. They had both been plenty busy with the things they were doing in the years leading up to their meeting, so, unusual as it was, the timing was simply perfect.

I've been told that in the tropics this concept is sometimes called *coconut time*. A coconut drops when it's ready to drop. We can't know when it will happen, but we can sure waste a whole lot of life force trying to figure it out. Sometimes the coconut drops and we can't figure out why it took so long. That's not our business, and we aren't served by making it our business. Life is going on, and it's up to us to go on with it.

My father used to tell us a story that demonstrates this well. One day, he and our dear family friend Harry Dean were sent out to kill a crocodile. Every so often, they would be asked to kill what we called a "man-eater"—an older predator that had become too slow to hunt as usual, who had gotten the taste of humans and figured out they were easy prey. Those animals would stalk villages, sometimes killing entire families one by one. Harry and my dad were known to be brave, rugged, and good shots, so when they got word of those animals, they would go out to kill them as quickly and humanely as they could.

Well, they located and killed the crocodile and then started to process the carcass to make the most they could of it. Inside the croc's stomach, they first found piles of jewelry. That was both horrifying and relieving because it meant they'd gotten the right one: the crocodile had eaten at least one well-to-do lady. As they were picking through the muck in its stomach, they found something else: a turtle. It had turned stark white from the time it had spent covered in the acidic contents of the crocodile's stomach. My father and Harry marveled at the sight.

Then something even more shocking happened: the turtle began to move. It stretched its head out of its shell—slowly, as turtles do—rose to its feet, and lumbered away.

My father told us that story over and over when we were kids. We loved it, and he swore it was true. "Imagine it from the turtle's perspective!" he would crow. "He sure didn't foresee a rescue! When things look dark and you're tempted to give up, remember the turtle and hang on a little longer."

As kids, we learned to hang on. I thought of that turtle often as I went through the harder moments in my life, the times that felt as dark as the inside of a crocodile's belly. I also thought of that turtle when there were aspects of universal timing that I simply couldn't understand. Everything takes its own time—it simply isn't up to us to understand it.

Healing, too, takes its own time. More often than not, time is the secret ingredient that allows healing to take place.

Sometimes, while we're wishing things would hurry up, they're doing exactly what they should be doing. If we weren't so bent on making everything go faster, it might be easier to embrace femifesting as it takes place.

Understanding this opens us to a new possibility—one we may not have considered before. What if the longer things take, the better they are? What would that mean? What if, instead of chasing youth and lost time, we could embrace the aging process, making space for our lives to get better and better as they go along?

Consider this radical concept: contrary to what our youth-obsessed culture might have us believe, we can actually become *better* as our bodies grow older. In fact, we should!

When seen from this perspective, growing older is no longer about compensating for lost or weakened capacities but rather about getting closer to embracing who we are meant to be. Each year that goes by connects us more to our purpose.

I had another chance to learn that when I found my voice at ninety-three.

I dreamed that I was a child and had sneaked away to sing nonreligious songs on a Sunday. That was looked down upon in my home so I was worried that I'd get into trouble for it. But then Jesus himself appeared and laughed, encouraging me to keep singing anyway. I woke up with a jolt.

At that point, I'd been a doctor and medical leader for many decades. I was a mother and grandmother and a great-grandmother, too. I had been using my voice for some time. I'd treated patients, spoken at conferences, sung lullabies. Yet I hadn't learned to trust my own voice. I hadn't learned to trust my intuition regarding what I knew to be true: in this case, that singing was *always* a good thing if it was done with joy! After more than nine decades on the planet, I still continued to doubt that my message was good enough or that I had what it took to adequately express it.

If I hadn't had that dream and found my voice, perhaps I wouldn't be writing this book to you today. That was the time it took for me to get to this moment.

My father surely didn't know how the last few years of his life would go. At first, after my mother died, we were all worried about what he would do with himself. The two had been such a team for so long. They had more than a marriage; they were colleagues, friends, confidants. They had lived unusual lives, which may have made it hard for him to relate to others who had chosen a more conventional path. I didn't want him to be lonely.

Then my father did something that surprised us all. He first became friends with my sister-in-law's mother, whom we all called Mother Daniels, and then he suddenly announced that they were going to get married. We all thought that was simply delightful. My nephew, who was already in medical school, got to have fun with it; he had to get permission from his professors to take time off and attend the wedding, so he told them he was going to see his grandparents get married. They answered, "Well, do you think it's about time?"

During the years my parents were together, there had been a lot of joy but also a lot of work. They were on a mission, quite literally. Mother Daniels's first marriage had been similar: strong, secure, solid. But my father and Mother Daniels decided that their marriage would be different. They were still companions, but they put the focus on fun, without any hard work involved. Both felt that they had never really played in their lives. In his final two years, she quilted and he played chess. They simply had fun together.

When my father knew he was reaching the end, he told Mother Daniels that he wanted to be buried with my mother, and she understood. They flew down to Arizona, and he went straight to the hospital, where he stayed until he died. Mother Daniels sang him hymns while he made the transition. With his dying breath, he mouthed the words along with her. On the drive home that day, Mother Daniels and I talked about the *Hallelujah!* everyone was singing on the other side. We marveled at the sweet beauty of Mother Daniels releasing my father to my mother, who would welcome him in the next realm.

After a long and happy marriage to my mother, those years with Mother Daniels were the icing on his cake.

I'm pleased to tell you that the most recent few years of my life have been absolutely marvelous. My family has grown. I've come to learn more about myself. And I'm not finished yet. In fact, I still wake up with the same thought I have every morning: "Okay. What are we going to learn today?"

Learning helps us reach for what's next—and reaching for what's next helps us come alive.

One of the ways to keep reaching for what's next is to make a ten-year plan. Why a *ten*-year plan? Well, if we think about our entire lives, it's simply overwhelming. Likewise, if we focus on too small a span of time, we feel inept, as though we can't get anything done. You can do this right now. It's simple: get out a pen and paper, and write down what you want to do within the next decade.

A ten-year plan makes space for everything. It ensures that there will be time to femifest *and* to manifest. It's a far enough reach that it keeps our life force activated. Yet it's close enough that we can achieve it, dust ourselves off, and plan anew.

My current ten-year plan involves bringing a dream I've held for a long time to reality. Since the 1970s, I've been envisioning a Village for Living Medicine, where people can come together to practice wellness and be fully alive. It will be more than just a center for healing; it will be a true community, where human bodies are recognized as the divine sanctuaries that they are. The people in my village will not be at war with life but rather in love with it. In my village, we'll be reaching for life—together.

As you make your own plan, I encourage you to set clear goals while leaving plenty of room for mystery. Because we never know when things will suddenly change, when some stubborn thing will give way to something new.

We never know when we'll find ourselves spontaneously healed. We don't know when we'll be blessed with forgiveness or our dream will finally break through, manifesting itself in front of us.

All we know for certain is that something is happening, and we are an integral part of it.

Back in the lecture on husband-coached childbirth, I continued to silently counsel my child as Bill sat quietly beside me. He had no idea what was happening as my two hands cradled my belly. When the time felt right, I gently started to put pressure on my child's butt. I continued to coach him through the process all the while.

"Listen up, baby. I can help guide you, but I can't do it alone. You've got to move, now. Get your little butt up there! Put your head down; it's time to face life!"

Suddenly, I felt him release under my hand. In an instant, he turned over in my womb, flipping like a fish jumps from the water. He settled half a second later, head down, butt up. As my body adjusted to his new position, I leaned back and smiled.

Two weeks later, that child and I labored together. Surrounded by our loving family, I welcomed my son David into this marvelous, wonderful world.

It's my sincere hope that as you've read my words, they have resonated within you—or, if not, that they someday will. These are the greatest lessons I've learned in my 103 years. I offer them as gifts. May you receive them gladly.

Just as I turned my son, I've worked through these pages to turn you toward life. This is an ongoing process. It's a practice we must embrace over and over again. In it, we're called to radically, but gently, flip our understanding on its head, from thinking that *we are in life* to understanding that *life is in us.*

Perhaps your connection with life has faltered just a little. Perhaps you're struggling with the realities of the world as it is. Or perhaps you're like most of us, somewhere in between, bouncing between higher moments and lower moments and wanting to bring them all meaning. Whichever is your case, it isn't too late for you to turn toward the life force within you.

Whether you've never known it or you've simply forgotten, I promise that life is there, pulsing through your body and soul, waiting.

Acknowledgments

Near the end of writing this book, I had a dream.

I was at a gala where I was going to receive an award. Everyone was seated at round tables, and someone was presenting onstage. My table was near the back of the room. The person onstage introduced me and called me up to receive the award. I rose to my feet as everyone in the room turned to look at me and began to clap.

It was at that moment that I realized I was wearing a long dress with buttons running down the back from my neck to my waist. It was also at that moment that I realized the long line of buttons was undone.

I stood there in shock. How was I going to walk across that room with my buttons undone? I couldn't reach them, and it would take me too long to fit each button into its buttonhole even if I could. Everyone was watching and waiting for me to step onto that stage and do what I'd come to do.

Yet faith called me. Hope beckoned. Something deep and true, something beyond me, compelled me to begin walking anyway. So I did.

As I stepped forward from my table, I was surprised to feel someone reaching behind me to fasten the bottom button.

I walked a few steps farther and felt another set of fingers button the next one.

I kept walking as the people in the room clapped for me, and each one I passed fastened another button on my dress. By the time I got to the edge of the stage, I had been buttoned from bottom to top. I was relieved and grateful. I knew I could do what I had come to the gala to do: climb the steps, say a few words, smile, and accept the award I had earned.

But as the dream showed me, I couldn't do it alone. Perhaps none of us ever does it alone. Perhaps our greatest work is done in union, in connection to other people. At least, my life has certainly gone that way. Isn't that wonderful?

One by one, I offer my deepest gratitude to everyone who fastened a button so I could complete this book. It is through them that I could present this understanding to the world. It is only with their help that this book could come to be.

Thank you to my mother and dad, Dr. Beth Siehl Taylor and Dr. John C. Taylor, who taught me not only about unconditional love but also about its sacred role in medicine. I'm grateful to have been raised alongside three great brothers, John, Carl, and Gordon, and my beloved sister, Margaret, who remained my dearest friend until the day she died. To the best ayah in the world, and to her husband, Dar, who baked us all birthday cakes in an upside-down dishpan over the fire and taught me to love curry from the beginning. Thank you to the villagers, the children, and everyone who helped in the field camps, who showed me how a simple life could be a good life. I'm grateful to my aunt Belle, who reminded me to tough it out and keep the faith, and to Harry Dean, whose sense of adventure I have always admired. Thank you also to Miss McGee, who taught me how to read and even encouraged me through my teens and young adulthood. You all helped form a wonderful childhood that turned into a wonderful life.

To Jadwiga Kushner, my best friend in college, who sang like an angel, and Dr. Jacqui Chavalle, my college roommate from France, whose global view of life helped me feel less alone. I'm grateful to my aunts Lou, Clara, and Lydia, and the Siehl family in Cincinnati, who were such a source of support for Margaret and me as we went through college so far from our parents. I'm also thankful for Albert and Louise Hjerpe, without whom I would never have met Bill McGarey, and who became a wonderful aunt and uncle to me through marriage.

I am forever grateful to the best home helper I have known since Ayah, Mrs. Cain, who came to our rescue in Wellsville, and whose German view of housekeeping, bread baking, and stern child rearing enabled us all to make it through some of the busiest years I could imagine. Thank you to my brother- and sister-in-law John and Irma McGarey, who became dear friends. They owned the Tastee Freez, but as far as my kids were concerned, the biggest treat of all was the fact that they also owned a television. To their son, John B. McGarey, MA, who has been supportive both personally and professionally. To my other brother- and sister-in-law, Lieutenant Colonel Bob and Jane McGarey, who were always there when I needed them. And to my Wellsville colleagues Drs. Bill and Edith Gilmore, who stood by me during some very difficult times.

Lester and Billie Babcoke became longtime friends after we moved to Arizona, and they were the ones who introduced me to Edgar Cayce. I was and remain profoundly grateful to Edgar Cayce, whose teachings were so influential to my philosophy. I am proud to say that his son Hugh Lynn Cayce became a dear friend to whom I am also grateful. I appreciate the way Charles Thomas Cayce and Kevin Todeschi have kept Hugh Lynn's work alive and well. Thank you to Peter and Alice Riddle, who became part of our extended family in those years. And I have to say, all those who shared in my Association for Research and Enlightenment (ARE) "Search For God" study group year after year became lifelong friends as well. To Dr. Norman Shealy, Dr. Evarts Loomis, and Dr. Gerald Looney, who founded the American Holistic Medical Association (AHMA) one weekend in Hemet, California, along with Bill and me, and to the amazing people who came and went through the AHMA throughout the decades, I say thank you. And to all those who helped establish, coordinate, and attend the conferences and other events of the Academy of Parapsychology and Medicine. I couldn't possibly list them all, so I'll just offer my thanks to the multitude of incredible physicians who joined our paradigm shift that became holistic medicine. You know who you are.

The ARE Clinic was able to touch the lives of innumerable people, many of whom came to learn and left to share what they learned with the world at large. To the countless people who moved through the ARE Clinic as physicians, technicians, nurses, therapists, staff, patients, volunteers, and financial supporters, I am in deep heartfelt appreciation.

To my brother Carl and his organization Future Generations, which enabled me to do my international work. And to all those around the world who touched me, taught me, shaped me, and loved me over the years, again I say thanks.

To my faithful volunteer secretary of forty years, Grace Page, who never wavered in her steadfast devotion to keeping my vision alive, I send a hug to beyond the grave.

To those who worked on creating the Scottsdale Holistic Medical Group, especially George Andres, Reni Simon, and Joe Kalish, who helped us get up and running in two weeks, and my daughter Helene, who is the heart and soul of that amazing healing home to this day, I cannot find words adequate to express my appreciation. And to all those who worked there or passed through those doors, I am forever grateful.

To those who participated in the creation of the Beth Taylor Foundation, which became the Gladys Taylor McGarey Medical Foundation and today is called the Foundation for Living Medicine, and to those who have ever worked on the board of this wonderful organization; there are too many to list, but they all have my gratitude, especially Bobbie Woolf, Jerome Landau, Fern Stewart Welsh, Barbara Heinemann, and Rose Winters, without whose leadership the foundation would not be the incredible organization it is today.

To those who blessed us with their musical talent, I bow in respect—especially to Joyce Buekers, Steve Halpern, and Steve McCarty.

To those who always saw beyond the present and stood by me with their emotional, practical, pragmatic, spiritual, and financial support—especially Ann McCombs, Dianne Schumacher, Mary Ann Weiss, and Frances Tesner—I couldn't have done it without you.

Thank you to Dr. Katey Hauser, who has helped me reach others with my message through Instagram, and to John Marshall, who has kindly provided me with massage for decades. And to all those practitioners who learned from me and carried what I learned out into the world beyond: without all your efforts, mine wouldn't mean much more than a hill of beans.

To all those who led and attended the myriad conferences I participated in year after year after year—Council Grove and ARE Clinic Symposia, the Academy of Parapsychology and Medicine conferences, ARE Conferences at Asilomar, AIHM symposia, Therapeutic Touch Nurses Group Symposia, and so many others—I learned so much at each of these. I pray that others did as well.

To my many friends in Scottsdale and beyond, I value your love so highly: Mantosh Devji, Doris Solbrig, Rita Davenport, James Mc-Cready, Mimi Guineri, Marlene Summers, Linda Landau, Lindsey Wagner, and Dianne Ladd. And to everyone else I haven't mentioned, thank you.

I treasure the marriage I shared with Dr. Bill McGarey and don't regret one minute of it. I am deeply grateful for our years together, as I am for the freedom I claimed after we parted ways. Our time together was so important in my life, as well as the lives of many others; it fits perfectly into the greater whole.

Part of that greater whole includes the family we created. The morning after my 102nd birthday, I woke up to hear my kids downstairs and wondered, "Have I died and gone to Heaven?" But I guess I'm still alive, and these wonderful kids in their seventies are actually mine. I'm grateful to my six children and their partners: Dr. William "Carl" and Deedee McGarey, Reverend Dr. John and Reverend Dr. Bobbie McGarey, Analea McGarey, RPT, Robert McGarey, MA and Lia Nelson, Dr. Helene Wechsler and Nick Ligidakis, and Dr. David and Dr. Lee McGarey. Thank you to all my grandchildren: Gabriel Taylor, Julia McGarey, Timothy McGarey, John McGarey, Dr. Martha McGarey, Dr. Daniel Wechsler, Dr. Andrew Wechsler, Dr. Hannah Rabinovich, Jessica McGeverly, and David McGarey. I'm still learning every day from my twelve (and counting!) great-grandchildren, as well as from the newest great-great-grands who have begun to arrive.

This book would not have been born were it not for the drive of my agent, Douglas Abrams, who believed in me from the start. I offer gratitude to him as well as Rachel Neumann, Sarah Rainone, and everyone else at Idea Architects. I'm grateful to Jennifer Chan Tren, who played a pivotal role in helping my book find a home at Atria, and to Esme Schwall Weigand, whose early interviews and drafts helped me clarify my direction. Thank you to Michelle Herrera Mulligan, my editor at Atria Books, who took a chance on me, turned the format on its head, and made things even better. Thank you to Sarah Wright for her brilliant wordsmithing and Lynn Anderson for her attention to detail. An extra thank-you to my son John, who arranged it all. And thank you to Kathryn Chandika Liedel, who was able to make sense of my words by seeing my soul first, then writing it all down.

To all my life challenges, which have been my teachers, and to all the wonderful moments that gave me the juice to face them: thank you. I believe there are more beautiful moments to come.

Notes

1. Aliya Alimujiang et al., "Association Between Life Purpose and Mortality Among US Adults Older than 50 Years," *JAMA Network Open* 2, no. 5 (May 24, 2019): e194270, https://doi.org/10.1001/jamanetworkopen.2019.4270.

2. Randy Cohen, Chirag Bavishi, and Alan Rozanski, "Purpose in Life and Its Relationship to All-Cause Mortality and Cardiovascular Events: A Meta-analysis," *Psychosomatic Medicine* 78, no. 2 (February–March 2016): 122–33, https://doi.org/10.1097/psy.0000000000000274.

3. Patricia A. Boyle et al., "Effect of Purpose in Life on the Relation Between Alzheimer Disease Pathologic Changes on Cognitive Function in Advanced Age," *Archives of General Psychiatry* 69, no. 5 (May 2012): 499–504, https://doi.org/10.1001/archgenpsychiatry.2011.1487.

4. Elsevier, "Volunteerism: Doing Good Does You Good," *ScienceDaily*, June 11, 2020, www.sciencedaily.com/releases/2020/06/200611094136.htm.

5. Yogini V. Chudasama, Kamlesh K. Khunti, Francesco Zaccardi, Alex V. Rowlands, Thomas Yates, Clare L. Gillies, Melanie J. Davies, and Nafeesa N. Dhalwani, "Physical Activity, Multimorbidity, and Life Expectancy: A UK Biobank Longitudinal Study." *BMC Med* 17, 108 (2019), https://doi.org/10.1186/s12916-019-1339-0.

6. Buettner, Dan, "Power 9: Reverse Engineering Longevity," Blue Zones, https://www.bluezones.com/2016/11/power-9/.

7. Ashish Sharma, Vishal Madaan, and Frederick D. Petty, "Exercise for Mental Health" (letter to the editor), *Primary Care Companion to the Journal of Clinical Psychiatry* 8, no. 2 (April 2006): 106, https://www.ncbi.nlm.nih.gov/pmc/articles/.

8. Laura Mandolesi et al., "Effects of Physical Exercise on Cognitive Functioning and Wellbeing: Biological and Psychological Benefits," *Frontiers in Psychology* 9 (April 2018): article 509, https://doi.org/10.3389/fpsyg.2018.00509.

9. Lucas V. Lima, Thiago S. S. Abner, and Kathleen A. Sluka, "Does Exercise Increase or Decrease Pain? Central Mechanisms Underlying These Two Phenomena," *Journal of Physiology* 595, no. 13 (July 2017): 4141–50, https://doi.org/10.1113/jp273355.

10. Elizabeth Blackburn and Elissa Epel, *The Telomere Effect: A Revolutionary Approach to Living Younger, Healthier, Longer* (New York: Grand Central Publishing, 2017).

11. Daniel L. Surkalim et al., "The Prevalence of Loneliness Across 113 Countries: Systematic Review and Meta-Analysis," *BMJ*, February 9, 2022, e067068, https://doi.org/10.1136/bmj-2021-067068.

12. Julianne Holt Lunstad, "The Potential Public Health Relevance of Social Isolation and Loneliness: Prevalence, Epidemiology, and Risk Factors," *Public Policy & Aging Report* 27, no. 4 (2017): 127–30, https://academic.oup.com/ppar/article/27/4/127/4782506.

13. Nicole K. Valtorta et al., "Loneliness, Social Isolation and Risk of Cardiovascular Disease in the English Longitudinal Study of Ageing," *European Journal of Preventive Cardiology* 25, no. 13 (September 2018): 1387–96, https://doi.org/10.1177/2047487318792696.

14. Ashton Applewhite, *This Chair Rocks: A Manifesto Against Ageism* (reprint) (New York: Celadon Books, 2020).

15. Timothy W. Smith, Carolynne E. Baron, and Catherine M. Caska, "On Marriage and the Heart: Models, Methods, and Mechanisms in the Study of Close Relationships and Cardiovascular Disease," in *Interpersonal Relationships and Health: Social and Clinical Psychological Mechanisms*, eds. Christopher R. Agnew and Susan C. South (New York: Oxford University Press, 2014), 34–70, https://doi.org/10.1093/acprof:oso/9780199936632.003.0003.

16. Liz Mineo, "Good Genes Are Nice, but Joy Is Better," *The Harvard Gazette*, April 11, 2017, https://news.harvard.edu/gazette/story/2017/04/over-nearly-80-years-harvard-study-has-been-showing-how-to-live-a-healthy-and-happy-life/.

17. Elizabeth D. Kirby et al., "Acute Stress Enhances Adult Rat Hippocampal Neurogenesis and Activation of Newborn Neurons via Secreted Astrocytic FGF2," eLife, April 16, 2013, https://doi.org/10.7554/elife.00362.

18. Michael W. Stroud et al., "The Relation Between Pain Beliefs, Negative Thoughts, and Psychosocial Functioning in Chronic Pain Patients," *Pain* 84, no. 2 (February 2000): 347–52, https://doi.org/10.1016/s0304-3959(99)00226-2.

19. Gunnar Kaati et al., "Transgenerational Response to Nutrition, Early Life

Circumstances and Longevity," *European Journal of Human Genetics* 15 (April 25, 2007): 784–90, https://doi.org/10.1038/sj.ejhg.5201832.

20. Jonas Hilty et al., "Plant Growth: The What, the How, and the Why," *New Phytologist* 232, no. 1 (October 2021): 25–41, https://doi.org/10.1111/nph.17610.

About the Author

D̲r. Gladys McGarey, MD, MD(H), was born in 1920 and is internationally recognized as the Mother of Holistic Medicine. As a founding diplomate of the American Board of Holistic Medicine, she has had a family practice for more than seventy years, through which time she has tirelessly championed holistic medicine, natural birthing, and the physician-patient partnership. She is the cofounder and past president of the American Holistic Medical Association (now called the Academy of Integrative Health and Medicine), cofounder of the Academy of Parapsychology and Medicine, and was one of the first Western doctors to regularly utilize acupuncture in the United States. Dr. Gladys was also an early advocate for home birth. Her innovations for natural birth include the Baby Buggy program, founded in 1978, which featured a fully equipped paramedical and emergency transport vehicle for home births, and pushed the Arizona hospital system to welcome partners into the delivery room.

In 1970, she cofounded the ARE Clinic in Scottsdale, Arizona, where she pioneered the integration of allopathic and holistic medical practices, laying the groundwork for the cultural shift that recognizes alternative and holistic medical modalities. She also cofounded the Scottsdale Holistic Medical Group. Dr. Gladys's work continues through the Foundation for Living Medicine, a nonprofit that works to expand the knowledge and application of holistic principles through scientific research and education.

Dr. Gladys lives and works in Scottsdale, Arizona, where she has recently become a great-great-grandmother. She currently has a life consultation practice, maintains a healthy diet, and achieves a daily 3,800 steps with her walker. She rides a tricycle named Red Bird and enjoys a good piece of cake now and then.